HUSBAND-
COACHED
CHILDBIRTH

HUSBAND-COACHED
CHILDBIRTH

THE BRADLEY METHOD® OF NATURAL CHILDBIRTH

FIFTH EDITION

ROBERT A. BRADLEY, M.D.

Updated and expanded by
Marjie, Jay, and James Hathaway, AAHCC

BANTAM BOOKS

This book contains general information, ideas, and techniques that have been successfully used by many families to enhance their birth experiences. Please check with your own health care provider(s) and use your own good judgment in order to determine what information applies to your specific situation and which ideas and techniques are appropriate for you. Every situation is different. We make no guarantees or assurances of any kind to anyone. Only you can make the important decisions you will face during pregnancy, labor, and birth. The information in this book is presented in the hope that it will inspire you to seek the best and safest options for you, your baby, and your family.

HUSBAND-COACHED CHILDBIRTH
A Bantam Book
PUBLISHING HISTORY
Harper & Row hardcover edition published 1965
Bantam trade paperback revised edition / June 2008

For protection of the public, The Bradley Method and American Academy of Husband-Coached Childbirth have been registered in the United States Patent Office. Only those teachers currently affiliated (as listed on www.bradleybirth.com) with the American Academy of Husband-Coached Childbirth may teach The Bradley Method. For childbirth information contact: The Bradley Method, Box 5224, Sherman Oaks, California, 91413-5224, USA, or call (818) 788-6662
or toll-free (800) 4-A-BIRTH or visit the website:
www.bradleybirth.com.

Published by
Bantam Dell
A Division of Random House, Inc.
New York, New York

Cover design by Tom McKeveny

Book design by R. Bull

Library of Congress Cataloging-in-Publication Data
Bradley, Robert A.
Husband-coached childbirth : the Bradley method of natural childbirth / Robert A. Bradley ;
Updated and expanded by Marjie, Jay, and James Hathaway.—5th ed.
p. cm.
Includes index.
ISBN 978-0-553-38516-8 (trade pbk.)
1. Natural childbirth.   2. Natural childbirth—Coaching.   3. Husbands.   4. Fathers.
I. Hathaway, Marjie.   II. Hathaway, Jay.   III. Hathaway, James.   IV. Title.
RG661.B64 2008
618.4'5—dc22   2008005915

This book is dedicated to all mothers everywhere who give of themselves that others may live, and to the manager of my office, my home, and my life—my beloved wife, Martha, who symbolizes the true concept of motherhood, not only to her children but to all children.

—Robert A. Bradley, M.D.

CONTENTS

ACKNOWLEDGMENTS

This edition of *Husband-Coached Childbirth* has been made possible with the support and encouragement of Dr. Robert A. Bradley and Martha W. Bradley's daughters, Martha L. Krehely, Marianne V. Lindemann, and Susan L. Nelson, for the benefit of children around the world, who will be able to say, "Daddy helped born me."

Marjie, Jay, and James Hathaway

We, the daughters of Dr. Robert and Martha Bradley, would like to thank Marjie, Jay, and James Hathaway for the endless hours and continued effort that they tirelessly volunteered in updating this fifth edition of *Husband-Coached Childbirth*. Although you may notice that some of the text has changed, Dr. Bradley's message remains the same. We strive in his memory to enable the parents of today and tomorrow so that they may be blessed with joyous birth-days!

With sincere appreciation,
Martha, Marianne, and Sue

PREFACE TO THE FIFTH EDITION

by Marjie Hathaway

Dr. Bradley told me many times about his being born at home on a farm. His mother gave birth to a large (eleven-pound) baby with his father and doctor present. After nursing her new son she got up and made tea for all of them.

Growing up on a farm gave Dr. Bradley opportunities to watch animals give birth and nurse their young. His father warned him to stay quiet and not disturb animals when they are giving birth. This was an experience that changed his life, watching animals give birth naturally with confidence and joy.

When Dr. Bradley went to medical school he found that human women gave birth in pain, which was confusing because that is not what he had learned from nature to expect. This spurred him on to train and teach pregnant nurses what he saw in the woods and on his family's farm. After he took on the role of doctor-coach, one mother expressed her joy by hugging and kissing him while still on the delivery table. Dr. Bradley realized that the father (who was out in the waiting room) was the one this mother should be hugging and kissing.

From that time on, Dr. Bradley included the husband on the

birth team. It soon became apparent that the husband added a special, much needed component to the birth. No one is better suited to help achieve a natural birth than a loving husband.

Because of this success Dr. Bradley was asked to write *Husband-Coached Childbirth,* which was first published in 1965. Through the years Jay and I have helped with revising editions and development of The Bradley Method worldwide. Today we are doing this revision along with James, who gives a younger perspective to the book so that moms can learn how to birth in a beautiful natural fashion with the added support of their husbands. Women learn the natural process of birth and men learn how to coach, encourage, support, and bond to this mother and baby, making a new family.

Jay and I were invited by Karen Osterlund, a friend and co-La Leche League leader, to a talk sponsored by La Leche League in 1965 in Los Angeles, California; Dr. Bradley was speaking about his new book *Husband-Coached Childbirth.* Dr. Bradley said some fascinating things that evening. First of all, he said that mothers do not need medication to give birth! I had given birth three times using medication and originally thought this was an outrageous statement. I interrupted Dr. Bradley and told him that was not possible. It hurt so much with the medication, how could anyone give birth without medication? Dr. Bradley calmly told me (and the audience) that women who learn how to give birth find that they know what to do and give birth on their own without drugs.

Next, Dr. Bradley said that a husband should be man enough to finish what he starts—pregnancy. Husbands need to learn how to help this mother during pregnancy, labor, birth, and forever. Yes, he should be in the delivery room. Well, I thought that was a good idea, but in 1965 it was not a common occurrence.

Then Dr. Bradley said that the mother should put the baby to breast immediately after birth to nurse. I was shocked. I said to Dr. Bradley that was impossible. I was so groggy after the delivery of my three medicated babies that I would have dropped them on the floor. Dr. Bradley calmly told the audience, and me, that the reason I was groggy was from the drugs and not the birth. He said I would find nursing right after birth to be possible, enjoyable, and a medical safety factor.

Then Dr. Bradley said that after nursing, his mothers sit up and, along with their husbands, have a glass of orange juice to celebrate the new addition to their family. Then they pose for a few pictures and walk out of the delivery room together. Again, I interrupted Dr. Bradley. "Wait a minute, did you say walk? How could a mother walk after birth?" I could remember being in pain and unable to walk comfortably for days or weeks after the birth of my children.

Dr. Bradley just smiled and said again that mothers without drugs happily walk, after they nurse and have their orange juice, and love it. I was amazed. Now to top this off, Dr. Bradley said his patients went home two hours after giving birth! He added that he was there to take care of things if a problem occurred and that rarely happened. He considered himself a medical lifeguard, watching, waiting, and staying out of the way when things were going well. He said he was there to manage any abnormality or complication while the parents were expected to know how to manage normality and birth. His philosophy was the opposite from many doctors today, who will tell you they practice "active management."

When we went to this talk I asked him if he would take care of me if I flew out to Denver, and he said he would if we came to Denver six weeks before my due date. I said that was not possible, and he said how about four weeks, and I said no, and jokingly he said, "If I see you . . ."

Dr. Bradley's talk changed our lives. We went home and talked and talked. What we came up with was that Dr. Bradley's "husband-coached childbirth" method could not be worse than the medicated births I had already gone through. So I went to my doctor and told him all the things I wanted to do. I wanted no drugs, my husband present, immediate breast-feeding, walking, going home soon after birth. He said I was crazy and told me no woman could give birth without drugs. He did not agree with anything I had said. I went home and we talked and talked again.

The next day I started searching around Southern California for a doctor or hospital that would just allow my husband into the delivery room. I felt that if I got that much, I could eventually get the rest. After a couple of weeks, I was unable to find anyone willing to cooperate. I was very sad, but for the safety of my baby I resigned myself to another "knock 'em out, drag 'em out" delivery (as Dr. Bradley called them). I kept going to my doctor. I remember going to him on a Friday close to my due date. He checked me and said I was four centimeters dilated, he stripped my membranes and told me (as a matter of fact) that I would have my baby that weekend. I went home and, to my surprise, Monday morning I woke up and was still pregnant. We realized the doctor was wrong. Tuesday morning I woke up, still pregnant, and turned to Jay and said, "Let's go." With three kids in tow, we went to Los Angeles International Airport and got on a plane to Denver, Colorado.

Two days later we gave birth to our son James in Denver and I had no drugs! Jay was with me the whole time, I nursed, I walked out of the delivery room and instead of flying home two hours later, we went sightseeing instead. Today James helps us run the American Academy of Husband-Coached Childbirth (The Bradley Method), which enables Jay and I to travel to spread the word. Dr. Bradley asked that I not return to Denver every time I had a baby, instead go back to California and get things started.

When I returned home, I found other women who wanted the same experience. I started teaching classes. I did have to convince a hospital administrator that a woman in labor needs a coach. He agreed. But when my first couple arrived in labor, I got a call from him telling me that labor and delivery was no place for a father. I reminded him that he said that we could train a coach for a woman in labor, and this dad went to classes, read books, and practiced labor rehearsals. He was a trained labor coach and important support. The administrator agreed and we got our first "husband-coach" at a birth.

It was a gradual process but after many phone calls and requests to doctors and hospitals, asking about getting husbands into delivery rooms, most hospitals today worldwide include the father as an important part of the birth of his child.

As we developed a curriculum for Bradley classes, I felt a need for a way to show couples that birth was beautiful and joyful. Remember that in the late 1960s almost everybody believed the medical myth that husbands did not belong at birth and birth was beyond painful and awful. I asked my husband (Jay is a film producer with his own studio) to film the births of a few of my couples. We would then fly to Denver and show the film to Dr. Bradley. He was always thrilled we were doing this, and he would offer his comments about what we should add or change about the classes. His exercise teacher, Rhondda Hartman, was a great help with her ideas and suggestions. During this time frame Rhondda wrote *Exercises for True Natural Childbirth*. The classes grew and grew to the point where I was teaching more than I could handle. We started training other mothers who wanted to teach Bradley classes. In 1970 we had our first teacher training, thinking that one was all the world would need. Now we average fifteen workshops a year, with teachers in many other countries.

We have seen many childbirth methods come and go. Dr. Bradley simply told couples about the natural process that has worked for centuries. He advocated nutrition, exercise, education, relaxation, coaching, and feeling safe with someone who you want to be with you and protect you. What he taught is not complicated, just the simple truths, generation after generation. Through the years science has proved what Dr. Bradley observed (as a child on the farm): perspiring mammals giving birth.

Today with the help and support of experts in the field, The Bradley Method remains at the top in childbirth education, showing couples that the natural process works. This is proven by the continued growth in world population, and the experience of millions of women is an experience you, too, can share.

When Dr. Bradley passed away in 1998, we estimated that he and the growing method had directly affected more than half a million births. There is also the indirect effect of millions and millions of dads who were (and are) there to work as a team with the mother sharing the birth, and bonding when their baby is born. Dr. Bradley used to tell these dads: "Your child will say, 'My daddy helped born me.'"

This book is simply an update of the basic principles of natural childbirth that worked for Dr. Bradley, The Bradley Method, and ourselves. With each new edition this book has remained steadfast in value because of Dr. Bradley's vision of the natural process. He wrote about his own experience using common sense that people could understand. Today, evidence-based studies keep proving that he was right. Couples all over the world have confirmed that the natural process has worked for them. Bradley teachers throughout the world have shared this method based on Dr. Bradley's childhood observations of perspiring mammals. The natural process has worked for countless generations. We hope you enjoy it.

PREFACE TO THE FOURTH EDITION

by Robert A. Bradley, M.D.

Many years ago, Thomas A. Edison stated: "The doctor of the future will give no drugs but will interest his patients in the care of the human frame, in diet, and in the cause and prevention of human disease."

This happy future has arrived, and today we have a new awakening of what is referred to as "holistic" medicine.

Natural childbirth, with its humanistic, undrugged approach to parenthood, is the epitome of holistic medicine. When I entered the practice of obstetrics in 1947, many mothers were restrained in large cribs and wore football helmets to protect their heads from banging against the bars during wild antics induced by powerful drugs.

This "knock 'em out, drag 'em out" era of "deliveries" under drugs has, thank God, changed to the peaceful husband-coached picture of true natural childbirth. Using The Bradley Method classes and through prenatal training, mothers and fathers learn to follow nature and, as other mammals do, give birth without the terrible indignities of drugs. As Edison so astutely predicted, today's parents are instructed in caring for the human frame, in proper diet, and in the causes and prevention of complications of pregnancy.

The result is undrugged, clear-brained, intelligent "Bradley babies." These babies will solve the problems of the future with brains unaffected by drugs at birth.

Abstaining from drugs during known pregnancy, however, cannot be the total solution to drug-free pregnancies, since a woman can be as much as two weeks pregnant before a missed menstrual period signals pregnancy. If her customary life habits include over-the-counter drugs, caffeine, nicotine (from either primary or secondary smoking), alcohol, aspirin, antihistamines for allergies, etc., the tiny, newly growing baby will be affected by both the residual drugs in her body and what she currently may be taking.

This applies equally to the father of the baby. In this first two weeks of life, the fetus or embryo is at the most sensitive part of its development and should not be exposed to any chemicals foreign to the body.

It behooves all young fertile couples, the man included, to live a drug-free existence in case pregnancy occurs. This revision of *Husband-Coached Childbirth* is aimed at teaching both men and women how to birth as a team and to adjust to the stresses of life. I first proposed these principles in 1947 and published the first edition in 1965.

These principles are truly God's method and have been tested from ancient times through the present.

FOREWORD

Human beings usually give birth to one child at a time. It takes around nine lunar months from conception to the birth of a child. Hence, the preservation of the human species for the two million or so years that man has been on this earth has always been a dear thing. It is therefore understandable that pregnancy and especially the birth of a child should have been invested with special value, as witnessed by the customs, ceremonials, rituals, and other practices with which these events are associated in all societies.

In every human society, the birth of a child has been welcomed as the dramatic event it is, the unifying event that binds husband and wife and children together as no other event in the life of a family can. This was still the case even in the technologically advanced societies of the West in which, in the earlier part of the twentieth century, the child was usually born at home with a midwife assisting. In the warm and familiar ambience of the home, the whole family could be involved in the birth of the child, and quite often it was the husband who assisted at the delivery, whether he was prepared to do so or not.

But with the increasing shift to the hospital delivery room in which to have the baby—and 96 percent of our women now have their babies in hospitals—the birth of a baby became a mechanical routine, and no longer a matter of family participation. Unfortunately, we—especially in the United States—have become increasingly mechanized, so that today we feel very strongly that if we can take anything out of human hands and especially out of the human heart and put it through a machine, we have made progress. Indeed, we flatter ourselves that we can make machines that think like human beings, while not always pausing to reflect that in the process we have also succeeded in making millions of human beings who can feel and think like machines. It is a sorry reflection.

A hospital is a splendid place, but it is not, in my view, a place in which the most beautiful celebration in the history of a family, the welcoming of a new member into it, should occur. That event should be celebrated where it belongs, in the bosom of the family, in the home. Dr. Bradley, in this admirable book, does not quite agree. I am fully aware of the grounds of his disagreement, and I respect them, but on that point I believe this is no place to argue. I shall be producing a book on that subject in the future, and I shall be content to leave it to the future to arbitrate between us. But on virtually every other point I am in full agreement with Dr. Bradley, and I believe his book to be one of the most important contributions to the rehumanization of obstetrical practice that has been published in the twentieth century. If we can't yet have babies at home, the next best thing is to bring the home into the hospital. Something of this I attempted to do in proposing the idea of rooming-in more than fifty years ago. (A. Montagu, "Some Factors in Family Cohesion," *Psychiatry,* 1944.) Toward this end Dr. Bradley has made a monumentally important step in the right direction by bringing the father into the whole program of preparation for birth. It is not merely the revolutionary advance of having the father present during his wife's labor and the birth of their child in the "delivery room," but the sharing, insofar as that is possible for the male, of the pregnancy with his wife during the whole nine months thereof.

Dr. Bradley is concerned with restoring something of the ease and happiness, the security and the bountifulness as a human experience of pregnancy and birth to mother, father, and children. He requires no special understanding of technical terms—he explains them all, hardly ever resorting to a single one, in a breezy vernacular style that will endear him to all mothers and fathers. What Dr. Bradley is interested in is making the birth of a baby an experience that mother and father can look forward to with pleasure, experience with joy, and make the foundation of an ever-firmer bond between them.

Dr. Bradley is an experienced and thoroughly reliable guide. He is a pioneer, and this is a pioneer book. The mothers and fathers who will read it will feel like pioneers, too, if, as I hope, they decide to adopt and follow Dr. Bradley's recommendations, for they will be pioneering in the most important of all frontiers: the making of good human beings in a good family.

The family is the basis of society. As the family is, so is the society, and it is human beings who make a family—not the quantity of them, but the quality of them. As a contribution toward improving the quality of the family, Dr. Bradley's book is of major importance. It brings that institution down from the abstract level of sociological discussion to the firm ground of what one does in order to make the meaning of a word achieve the action it produces. In other words, this is a beautifully practical book that potential parents can use as the compass by which to steer their way into the safe harbor of happily born children in a happy family where everyone is given the opportunity to inherit his birthright, which is development—without the obfuscating and damaging effects of outmoded and wrongheaded traditional obstetrics.

—Ashley Montagu, Ph.D.

1

INTRODUCTION

The administrator of Porter Memorial Hospital in Denver, Colorado, called our office one day in 1961. He had received a request from the Canadian Broadcasting Corporation for permission to film a documentary on husband-coached natural childbirth for presentation on their program, *This Hour Has Seven Days*.

Mrs. Merle Grosman, of Toronto, a natural-childbirth mother herself and a member of the Natural Childbirth Association at the time, had initiated the idea and written to ask if we had patients who would cooperate.

In discussing it with her, we decided to utilize a woman having her first baby. There is a misconception promoted by the unknowing that having a baby by natural childbirth might be possible after having had other babies, but not with the first!

Accordingly we contacted our due or overdue primigravidas (women experiencing their first pregnancies), and after Tom Koch, director, and his crew of cameramen arrived, these women were photographed with their husbands at class, doing prenatal exercises, etc., as participants in mental and physical preparation for childbirth. Then everyone waited patiently for one of them to go into labor.

The law of the perversity of nature in general and pregnant women in particular manifested itself in that we had had many births just before our Canadian visitors arrived, then had to wait a week before one went into labor. This served to illustrate again that babies cannot read calendars and that doctors cannot tell when labor will begin.

As an honorary life member of the Toronto Natural Childbirth Association I was very much honored to be chosen to illustrate the great principles involved. I was also embarrassed that it took so long before a patient went into labor. I was bound by medical principles not to interfere with the development of a baby by forcing or inducing labor for anyone's convenience, so everyone waited.

Finally at midnight one night the phone rang, and Patricia and Gary Petersen announced they were on their way to the hospital. They were met at the hospital entrance by the somewhat sleepy but efficient TV camera crew of the CBC, who carefully followed the course of labor and birth with cameras and sound recorders. The visitors were intrigued and delighted by the calm self-assurance of these two young people who confidently went about the happy business of bearing a child as they had each been trained to do.

The husband had signed in for his wife while the nurse in attendance had performed the prep. He then joined his wife, to remain with her throughout labor and birth and share the requested privilege of walking back with her from the delivery room.

Their happy chatter as they strolled together in the early stages of labor would be rhythmically interrupted by uterine contractions. As her labor picked up in intensity they returned to the labor room and concentrated on their respective tasks. The old term "labor pains" just couldn't properly be applied here, for the observers could see no evidence of pain. The husband busily cranked the bed flat, arranged an extra pillow under his wife's raised knee as she turned on her side and assumed the "running" position of early first-stage labor that she had learned in class.

During the contractions the young mother would calmly lie curled up, peacefully close her eyes, and automatically relax all the muscles of her body. The young husband tenderly placed a guiding hand on his wife's abdomen and directed her diaphragmatic breathing. He would also lean over and maintain a constant soft whispering in his wife's ear during this interval.

The observing guests could not make out his words, but the endearing tone of his voice made apparent that the content was indeed the repetitious love "gobbledygook" with which she was so familiar. In prenatal classes the husbands are instructed to repeat verbally during contractions the intimate "love line" that was so effective in the moonlight originally and started the chain of events leading to the pregnancy.

When the muscle contractions of the uterus subsided, the chatter resumed, to be momentarily interrupted again as the uterus went about its work uninhibited. Between contractions he would rhythmically massage his wife's low back "saddle" area, accompanied by murmurs of approval from her. Whenever a contraction occurred, the same calm pattern of relaxation, abdominal breathing, and love talk would be automatically repeated.

As time went on, the husband occasionally slipped ice chips into his wife's mouth with a spoon to counter the drying effect of mouth breathing, which is part of total relaxation during contractions. The couple performed their respective tasks calmly, automatically, with light chatter between contractions. The observers from Toronto were impressed by the obvious fact that here were two people working happily together. Each knew, without being told, exactly what they were about.

As time went on, the interval between contractions gradually became shorter, the chatter accordingly gradually diminished, and the parents concentrated more and more on their respective tasks. Each said, when asked later, that they completely forgot about the presence of the observers; they were too busy.

The idea of some sort of medication being utilized in such an efficient, peaceful performance never occurred to the performers and seemed ludicrous to the observers. The close relationship between husband and wife, the total dependence upon each other, was heartwarming to see—that it truly "takes two to tango" was never more manifest. Again, the obvious ego-deflating question was put to me as the obstetrician: "Who needs a doctor for this?"

My occasional vaginal examinations to determine the dilatation of the cervix constituted rather rude interruptions that momentarily disrupted the smooth working pattern of the process. They obviously got along better when the doctor wasn't around. I answered their question by stressing again that the doctor's role is vital only when complications occur. Comparing birthing to swimming, the doctor is the lifeguard. Both swimming and birthing carry an irreducible minimal risk, and lifeguards and doctors are necessary, but only for complications. Good swimmers and good birthers need them to be present, but just in case problems arise.

As labor progressed, the parents became oblivious to everything and everyone as they carefully concentrated on the job at hand. This concentration was enhanced by the quiet, hushed "bedroom" atmosphere that is maintained in the labor rooms of this hospital. The importance of such an atmosphere is stressed as part of nurses' training in a course on the principles of natural childbirth.

Labor is what the term implies, hard work, and although mothers are trained to deliberately relax all muscles during uterine contractions, the uterus is of sufficient size and power as a muscular organ to produce perspiration in the mother in the later stages of labor. The husband's role included getting a cool washcloth and applying it tenderly to the perspiring brow of his wife. Such seemingly trivial acts reduce the tasks of nurses and direct the gratitude of a mother to the one she loves . . . her husband.

Between contractions, at the wife's request, the husband would alter her position occasionally by adjusting the bed so that she was half-sitting, with two pillows under her arms. Again, the familiar talk and cooperation would be evident.

The labor progressed to the transition stage, and the husband gently encouraged the techniques associated with this stage, knowing the need for change. The young mother shortly announced the urge to push, ushering in the second stage of labor. After a short vaginal check to verify the complete opening of the cervix, the husband adjusted the pillows behind his wife's shoulders and coached her in assuming the squatting position in the elevated bed. With the beginning of each contraction the mother would take two breaths and exhale them, waiting for the contraction to build in intensity.

This was followed by breath-holding and the expulsive pushing with contractions. After a few pushes in bed, the husband, doctor, and observers changed into scrub suits, caps, and masks while the attending nurses wheeled the mother to the nearby birth room.

The husband took his place at the head of the birth-room bed on what I call the "daddy stool," which prior to natural childbirth was occupied by an anesthetist. He resumed his coaching and adjusted the supporting pillows during each contraction to fit the contours of his wife's shoulders and back as she calmly held her breath, curled forward, and pulled her knees back under her armpits in the squatting position on the downward-tilted birth bed.

This position served to open wide the soft tissues of the birth canal to allow gradual descent of the infant. Because of the degree of additional exertion required of the mother in this stage, the husband utilized the cold, moist washcloth, not only to wipe away perspiration from her brow, but to have his wife bite on between contractions to maintain moisture on her lips, as he had been trained to do.

In this, the second stage, the infant had passed from the uterus into the vaginal canal, and the uterus now slowed down in the frequency of contractions with longer intervals between. This resulted in a return of the chatter between wife and husband. The observers were again impressed by the calm, peaceful attitude of the parents as they conversed between contractions about whether the baby would be a girl or a boy, and eagerly looked forward to knowing soon. The husband made an admiring comment on his wife's ability to hold her breath during contractions.

As the baby passed into the world, announcing her arrival with a lusty yell, the mutual exclamations of delight, "It's a girl!" by husband and wife, their shiny-eyed wonder at the miracle of this new life, and their mutual pride in accomplishment made a picture of wholesome togetherness bordering on ecstasy.

I then handed the infant to the mother to hold. This first real meeting with her child was accompanied by such a delighted, joyous expression on the mother's face that the husband, ready with his camera, recorded this important moment as a permanent record for the baby book.

The umbilical cord was later clamped and cut while the mother was holding the baby. The baby was then put at the mother's side for the first introduction to breast-feeding. The purpose of this from an obstetrician's point of view was not primarily nourishment, but to activate the reflex that stimulates uterine contractions to separate the placenta and decrease bleeding from the placental site. This is a safety factor for the mother and baby.

Breast-feeding also provides nourishment and this first feeding of colostrum, which provides immunities for the baby to keep it safe in its new environment. The colostrum starts the production of vitamin K in the baby's gut, building up to a peak at the eighth day and is important for blood clotting. Colostrum also acts as a laxative to get the baby passing meconium, which cleans the bowels out, reducing problems with jaundice. Having the baby at the breast, close and skin to skin, intensifies bonding between mother, father, and baby.

During this period of handling and nursing the child, husband and wife literally had their heads together. Their constant "parent talk" to the baby, calling her by name—Kirsten Lynn—and expressions of delight to each other were accompanied by intimate indications of mutual love, which made all the attendants feel like intruders.

The parents were playing with the baby, absorbed in counting fingers and toes, commenting on whose hair color she inherited, and so forth.

Each parent was then given a celebratory glass of iced orange juice—for the mother to replenish blood sugar, depleted from its utilization by the uterus, and to correct the drying effect of mouth breathing during labor. Orange juice also helps replace fluids lost during the birth process and provides sodium for fluid balance and potassium to prevent dizziness. The father is also given a glass of orange juice as a token of appreciation for his important participation and to maintain the great principle of sharing all aspects of this beautiful experience with his wife.

We joyfully refer to the orange juice as refreshment served at the original birthday party—which is the best of all birthday parties; the others are just pale substitutes for the real thing. Besides, only naturally born babies can accurately celebrate true "birthdays," the others are more appropriately celebrating "delivery days"!

The mother then expressed the desire to walk back from the birth room. She was given her robe and slippers, and with the baby in one arm, a glass of orange juice in the other hand, and a beaming, proud husband alongside, she strolled happily out the door and down the hall—mission accomplished. A helpful nurse, using the husband's camera, took a final picture of this new family group.

Since 1917 as a natural baby myself, observing animals on the farm and as a teacher of natural childbirth, I have seen this happy series of events repeated thousands of times. To our visitors from Toronto it was a new and never-to-be-forgotten experience.

I was delighted to have our busy office hours interrupted a few hours later by the director and photographers, who stopped by to express their admiration and praise of the method, and their gratitude for the privilege of witnessing the birth. Most significant to me was that they had sent flowers to the new mother and were passing cigars around as enthusiastically as if each were the father of the baby! The spirit of joy and pride in accomplishment of a natural birth is indeed contagious.

THE THEORY OF NATURAL CHILDBIRTH

GROWING UP ON A FARM

To anyone like myself who grew up in God's great outdoors and witnessed the birth process in domesticated and non-domesticated animals, other than human, the inevitable questions are bound to arise: Why do all other animals peacefully and joyfully give birth unassisted? Why can't the human animal do this? What makes the difference?

Throughout my childhood I was fortunate enough to live on the outskirts of a small town in what amounted to a farming environment. We had a large barn that in the course of years was occupied by many domestic animals. We averaged from eight to ten cats, had horses, cows, goats, and a succession of dogs. In addition to these domestic animals, the open countryside adjacent to our place afforded the opportunity to observe many animals in the wild.

ANIMAL BIRTHING

The birth processes I witnessed in these many creatures showed no objective evidence of pain or suffering. The opposite was true: the animal mother's eyes were radiant with joy and happiness. I based my practice on this observation of all animals, but mostly perspiring mammals.

This was brought back to my awareness not long ago. A sheep rancher, female variety, from a neighboring state had heard that I was a natural-childbirth doctor, so she came to see me when she discovered her pregnancy.

I'll never forget her first visit. She was over six feet tall, dressed in the clothing of her trade—boots, Levi's, and Stetson hat. She stormed into the office with great strides, and loudly and firmly announced to our office receptionist, and all present in the reception room, that her husband had gotten her pregnant during the lambing season and, "I just decided then and there, if those dumb sheep can give birth to their young that easily, so can I. I'm just as smart as they are!" Let me assure you that after completion of our training course she was every bit as good as her word—she was indeed as smart as her sheep and a marvelous natural-childbirth mother.

ANIMAL VS HUMAN (PERSPIRING MAMMALS)

What, then, is the difference between human and other animals? Are their bodies made differently? As a matter of fact, they are remarkably similar. Cat and dog bodies are used in premedical anatomy studies due to the similarity of structures with identical name and function. Is it that they just can't experience pain? Following a natural-childbirth newspaper article, an indignant letter to the editor asserted cats can have kittens without pain because they cannot feel pain as human beings do. I've often wondered if that misguided lady had ever stepped on a cat's tail in a darkened room or rocked on a cat's paw with a rocking chair.

No, that's not an adequate explanation, for animals otherwise manifest pain when hurt.

Could it be that all other animals instinctively do something that keeps the birth process from hurting? Could it be that they have built-in know-how, called instinctual knowledge, and automatically do the right thing at the right time? Humans, apparently lacking this instinctual knowledge, do the wrong thing; and the wrong thing hurts and prolongs labor. Moreover, could it be possible in addition to instinct that animals in the wild have learned from seeing others of their own kind give birth and raise their young?

CHANGING FROM HOME BIRTHS TO HOSPITAL DELIVERIES

In the 1940s women were changing from home to hospital where they gave birth alone and thus birth became a mystery to the next generation. That is why we need childbirth classes today. This way families can learn what they missed.

INSTINCT VS EVOLUTION KNOWLEDGE

My mind mulled over this thing called animal instinct. What is it? No one knows, but there it is, and there it acts. Not only in labor and birth, but also in swimming, or knowing what to do in water. Human beings are the only animals I could think of who drown when dropped in deep water; all other animals I know or could remember from my youth know how to swim, and do so immediately and perfectly when immersed. Also, human animals are the only ones I know who need to take compasses along on hunting trips—so they can find their way back home! Many other animals have a "homing instinct"—you can't lose that cat even if you try! It will frequently get home before you.

Does that mean that we should curse our Creator because He apparently shortchanged us and "forgot" to give us this knowledge? No, we are really the superior animals, judging by the fact that when we visit the zoo we are on the outside of the cages and they are on the inside. God gave us a magnificent brain capable of abstract thinking, a high level of communicative ability, learning, retention, reasoning, and so forth.

The current theory of natural childbirth is that we should study the animals and by intelligent reasoning learn to do, through education, training, and practice, what they do by instinct. Or, to make a blunt comparison, a woman who doesn't know how to swim is given nine months' notice that she will be thrown in deep water. Let's assume that during that nine-month period she does not avail herself of classes where swimming is taught. This is as unreasoning as one who knows she is pregnant, does not know how to act in labor, and then during her nine months does not bother to attend classes in the conduct of labor. The results in both cases would be horrible to behold, particularly by someone who loves the participant.

IMPORTANCE OF NATURAL-CHILDBIRTH TRAINING

Natural-childbirth training displaces ignorance, superstition, fear, anxiety, and the resultant bodily tensions that are such obstacles in labor and in swimming. There is nothing more pleasurable to observe than an expert human swimmer frolicking in deep water. Similarly there is nothing more marvelous to behold than an expert, educated, trained human mother giving birth.

NATURAL VS MEDICATED

Is it really necessary for women to suffer so in labor? Do they really have to be delivered? Must they lose all human dignity and self-control in labor from the drunken effect of medication given in the vain attempt to make labor pain-free? Does medication really make labor pain-free? If the answer to the latter question is not perfectly clear in your mind, I beg you, ask women who have tried the medication method! They may tell you they could not have done it without the medication and everyone should take that epidural.

These women may be surprised that no drug, including the drugs in epidurals, have been proven safe for an unborn baby. For nine months women are warned to stay clear of all drugs in order to protect their baby, yet at the time of birth this is forgotten. Restaurants are actually required to post warnings to pregnant women about drinking alcohol. Remember couples need natural-childbirth training to know how to give birth and many medicated women don't know what they have missed or are capable of doing.

This brings to mind an article I read years ago, written by an intelligent career woman, a journalist, as I recall. She had married late in life after a brilliant career, deciding in the last few months of fertility that she wanted to become a mother before nature shut off this function. Being a strong-willed person, she acted upon her decision and became pregnant. Being also a scientifically oriented person, she enthusiastically investigated the next logical question: "What's it like, having a baby? What am I to expect?"

She found there were in existence two fundamental ways: One involved medication and anesthetics to relieve pain and being passively "delivered" of her baby. The other was the method of natural childbirth whose enthusiastic advocates disdained the "knock 'em out, drag 'em out" approach and actively gave birth to babies without any "pain relief" medication at all. She applied, sensibly, the old car slogan, "Ask the man who owns one."

She proceeded carefully to interview a group of mothers who had used the medicated method—"Between us girls, what was it really like to have a baby?" The answers were horrifying: "Natural birth did not work for me," "My body does not work," "I don't have time for classes." Many mothers said they loved their new baby and thanked the anesthesiologists for taking away the pain but: "Never again!" "Worst pain I have ever known!" "Most terrible experience of my life!" "I know it's my fault, but the pain in my back has never gone away."

Many of these mothers tell other women to take the epidural, how could you birth without it? Don't be a martyr, this is the twenty-first century. They all seem to believe, mistakenly, that these sophisticated, complicated drugs do not get to or affect their baby. These drugs do get to their unborn baby! Would they let their kindergartner have similar narcotics?

She then interviewed natural-childbirth mothers, and I heartily encourage any honest skeptic to do likewise. "It was wonderful!" "Most beautiful experience of my life!" "Why would anyone want to be asleep at such a wonderful moment?" "Giving birth was one of the most exciting, life-changing experiences of my life." "Experiencing natural childbirth has made me realize how powerful I am." "If I can birth, I can do anything."

One woman who had experienced both ways described it as the difference between being raped by a stranger and being loved by your husband. Some of the mothers used the term "birth climax," subjectively comparing the feeling of birth with the emotional/physical climax in lovemaking.

ANESTHESIA

Even today general anesthesia is still being used, as are spinals and epidurals. Some women get "walking epidurals" (combined spinal epidural, or CSE) or a combination of a spinal and an epidural along with the side effects of both. These procedures often use a cocktail of drugs that include narcotics such as lidocaine, morphine, fentanyl, and many, many others.

These drugs are addictive, painkilling, and mind altering, which some women feel as a thrilling high, and these drugs are controlled by the Food and Drug Administration. These drugs go to and affect the baby. Studies have been done where a drug is administrated to the mother, and then scalp vein samples are taken from the baby. The drug is found in the baby's blood in less than three minutes after giving it to the mother.

DRUGS AFFECT THE ABILITY TO BREAST-FEED

These drugs also affect the important natural process of breast-feeding. Because there is a fear that the mother might become nauseated and throw up, she is often given drugs to dry up the secretions in her stomach. These may also dry the secretions in her breasts making breast-feeding a challenge, often very difficult and sometimes impossible. Many women are so angry with the overuse of medication that they choose to have a home birth next time. Birth is hard work and sometimes painful but it can be the most rewarding experience of your life.

DR. BRADLEY'S SUCCESS HISTORY

After forty-six years and well over twenty-three thousand attended births by natural childbirth, I have often stated that the only handicap I have found in the method is the super enthusiasm of the parents afterward. They will talk your ear off and many of them have written or been featured in articles about natural childbirth.

This very book was written at the persistent insistence of my own patients, others, and Bradley teachers around the world who have experienced the joy of natural childbirth.

Back to the bewildered young doctor and former farmer. The theory sounded too simple, even oversimplified. But it might be true—maybe humans could imitate animals in labor and enjoy similar unmedicated births. But what is the scientific explanation? What is the mechanical and physiological action? I didn't know then, and I don't know now. I doubt if I'll ever know the academic explanation of why or how it works. However, being a clinician (one who does), I tried it out in 1947. I applied these principles, and, believe me, they do work.

Women can give birth by the action of their own bodies, as animals do. Women can enjoy the process of birth and add to their dignity by being educated to follow the example set by instinctive animals. Women can take joy and pleasure from the privilege of being women and bless God for being able to give birth, instead of showing snarling hostility toward the men who love them—because men don't have to have children.

3

"IT'S NOT NICE TO FOOL MOTHER NATURE"

PERSPIRING MAMMALS

In 1947, I first proposed the theory of true "natural" childbirth in humans, basing the mother's conduct upon exact imitation of the other mammals which, like ourselves, have perspiration glands. My attention was first directed this way by Dr. Grantly Dick-Read of England, but I was puzzled by some aspects of his method. He had his patients panting in labor, and I had never seen any animal pant, except the ones lacking perspiration glands, who used this odd method of breathing as a means of cooling their bodies. Mammals with perspiration glands simply don't breathe that way! Also, Dr. Dick-Read ignored the husband during labor, and he himself sat at the head of the bed so his patient could see him at all times. This was most impractical, as few practicing physicians worth their salt would have time to do this.

IMPORTANCE OF ACTIVE SUPPORT
BY THE HUSBAND

You will find, as you study this book, that the husband should be the one in constant attendance. Because of his love relationship with his wife, he is far more capable of achieving cooperation and helping her self-control than any attending doctor. We therefore call this approach "husband-coached" natural childbirth.

We may be assuming the best, but the chances are that this husband is also the father and has a vested interest in seeing his baby born. Today on television news we often see reports on what are called "Deadbeat Dads": men who have no interest in their children and refuse to pay child support even though these are their children. Some Deadbeat Dads are going to jail or having their salaries garnished because of this. How many of these men were there, trained, coaching at the birth, and active participants in the birth of their child(ren)?

Dr. Marshall Klaus, of the Department of Pediatrics, Case Western Reserve University School of Medicine, has done studies (*JAMA,* 1991) that show that mothers who have doulas (from a Greek word meaning a slave skilled in midwifery) or a labor assistant (I chose to use the husband) have shorter labors and are likely to receive less medication. I feel men make the best labor coaches because of their close, loving relationship with this woman and also with their baby.

OVERWHELMING SUCCESS RATE

Since the introduction of husbands along with training classes, my patients had 96 percent unmedicated births. I do realize that not all mothers choose to have husbands these days. They still need coaches, someone they can trust and someone with whom they can relate. They need someone who will come to class with them, encourage them when it comes to good nutrition, exercise with them, practice labor rehearsals, and be there anytime needed. Significant others, friends, family members, or paid support persons are all possible coaches for labor.

This is another wonderful trip into the past, since this is the way our ancestors celebrated birth, together as a family or extended family. These support people should be family or friends if at all possible.

If you are a non-husband coach, please forgive my old-fashioned way of referring to the husband as coach. The message is the same. Read *Assistant Coaches Manual* by Susan Bek, AAHCC, and Marjie Hathaway, AAHCC, available at www.bradleybirth.com.

NATURAL AS IN NATURE

The term "natural" implies the way it is done in nature, and anything that deviates from this cannot truly be called natural. Many Johnny-come-lately imitators have appeared in recent years, with a multitude of variations in breathing techniques with some rather odd activities to distract the mother from her uterine activity. Some groups have achieved the acceptance of doctors by stating that they are not trying to get the doctors to use fewer drugs and medications, rather, they are just trying to make childbirth "more meaningful," whatever on earth that means!

HAVE IT YOUR WAY BIRTHING

There has developed also what I sarcastically call "Burger King" obstetrics, after a hamburger chain that advertised "Have It Your Way," which encourages doing anything you wish in labor. Some books advocate changing the position the baby chooses or forcing the baby to come early. Such labors are usually long and gruesome; doing what is right (instructed labor) doesn't take anywhere near as long and is far more comfortable.

I remember a patient who had been taught this "any alternative you wish" approach in labor, then came to me and went into labor before we could train her in true natural childbirth. She found sitting bolt upright in late first-stage labor to be a little less uncomfortable, and insisted on sitting that way for two hours, remaining six centimeters dilated without change. In desperation, I gently suggested that she assume the "running position" on her side, which we teach in order to displace the uterus upward out of the pelvis to allow the cervix to dilate. I pointed out that sitting on her cervix created pressure that interfered with blood circulation and created numbness, but this also interfered with cervical dilatation and didn't produce a baby. A few contractions in nature's position resulted in complete dilatation and birth very shortly.

THE NATURAL PROCESS WORKS!

The purpose in all this is to have a baby, not seek comfort. It is true that the most comfort comes from doing something right, but this is achieved through learning what is right from experienced teachers before labor ensues, not frantically experimenting by yourself in labor. Remember the stronger the contraction the sooner the baby. You will learn in Bradley classes to welcome the strength of the contraction. It is for a purpose. Avoid these "any alternatives you wish" people and get back to nature. Our Creator knows not only what is best for other mammals but also what is best for human mothers. In His wisdom, He gave other mammals built-in know-how; He gave people speech and the ability to learn what is right through prenatal education.

May I earnestly implore couples contemplating childbirth not to accept these compromises. Anytime you deviate from the great principles of Mother Nature you are going to be sorry you did. There was a rather amusing TV commercial years ago in which a woman representing Mother Nature is tricked into thinking that a particular brand of margarine is true butter. She angrily states, "It's not nice to fool Mother Nature!" then, *Wham!* She causes a lightning bolt to strike. If you fool around with nonnatural ways of conduct, there are many "whams" you will suffer from, some obvious, some subtle, some known, and many yet to be discovered.

To motivate you into not only reading but studying the rest of this book, in order to achieve true natural childbirth, let's consider some of the "whams" that may follow if you don't.

WHAM ONE: THE ILL EFFECTS OF DRUGS AND MEDICATION ON THE BABY!

Other methods of childbirth state that "a little medication won't hurt anything." Natural-childbirth principles have always stated that our firm goal is totally unmedicated pregnancy, labor, and birth. We want pregnant women to avoid taking any form of drugs in any doses at all before or during pregnancy: aspirin, cold remedies, nicotine, alcohol, tonic water with quinine in it (it can cause deafness in the baby), inhaled hair spray, even food with preservatives (if bugs won't eat it, why do we have to?). The list of things to avoid grows constantly.

DRUGS NOT SAFE FOR DELIVERY

Women should be wary of all drugs. None of them have been proven safe in pregnancy. If you are taking a prescription medication, review it with you doctor/midwife, pediatrician, and pharmacist. Pharmacists today generally try to educate the patient about drugs they are taking, and how they react with other drugs and their side effects. Always weigh the risk versus the benefit of taking any drug. There may be times when a mother needs to take a drug. If she is having seizures or perhaps asthma and cannot breathe—these can be life threatening and are not good for the mother or baby. Discuss this with your doctor/midwife, pediatrician, and pharmacist. Ask if this is the right drug, the right dosage, and if you taking it for the correct amount of time.

Over-the-counter drugs have the same problem. They have never been proven to be safe in pregnancy. Aspirin can change the clotting properties of your blood. Tylenol can affect your liver. Read the label. Many people take more than the amount recommended. This can be a serious problem.

Think about why you need one of these drugs. Do you have a headache? Why? Is it because you have not eaten lately or perhaps you are dehydrated from lack of drinking water? Are you working too hard? Are you not getting enough sleep? Is stress in your life? Can you make changes in your lifestyle so that you do not get headaches? Healthy lifestyle changes can last a long time. Most drugs are for a short time and have to be taken over and over again.

SOCIAL DRUGS
Scary as it may sound there are many social drugs that may have ill effects on unborn babies. Alcohol has been proven to be a problem and today most restaurants and bars have posted signs about the danger of pregnant women drinking any alcohol. It can cause fetal alcohol syndrome with symptoms very much like Down syndrome.

SMOKING!
First- and secondhand smoke may endanger the unborn. When a mother inhales smoke, nicotine and other harmful agents get into her blood and go to the baby through the placenta. Tests have shown that the baby's heart may stop beating temporarily. When the baby is born you can see the nicotine's effect on the placenta. The placenta may have a yellow, dingy appearance.

WATER
Every year your local newspaper generally prints a warning from the federal government and state governments about being careful about the water you drink. If you drink city water that is processed with chlorine and that chlorine comes in contact with an organic substance, such as a leaf, it turns into trihalomethane, which increases the miscarriage rate by 50 percent.

Boil or Bottled?   It is recommended that you boil the water and leave it in an open container overnight in the refrigerator, or filter the water. You may want to drink bottled water, but you still need to read the label. Some waters put magnesium sulfate in the water. Magnesium sulfate is a powerful substance that is used to stop early labor, it is a muscle relaxant, athletes put it into bathwater and soak in it to relieve muscle aches, and it is used as a laxative. Ask the company that processes the water to send you a copy of the chemical analysis so you can read about what you are drinking.

FOODS
Read the labels. Some cereals have ingredients you may not know about, understand, or want to eat. One such ingredient is trisodium phosphate (TSP). It is a chemical that is used in heavy cleaning. Perhaps you don't want to eat it.

CAFFEINE
Caffeine comes in many forms: chocolate, coffee, sodas. The baby's blood-brain barrier (BBB) is immature and this caffeine is affecting your baby. When you drink a caffeine drink your blood-brain barrier tries to protect your brain, the baby's blood-brain barrier is incomplete so the effect of the caffeine may be greater on your baby than it is on you. Note that some of the drinks that are not caffeinated have phosphoric acid in them and that has been shown to leach the calcium out of your bones.

OTHER ITEMS
There are a lot of things to be careful of, red or yellow dye, (actually any color), MSG, nitrates, sugar, artificial sweeteners, cleaning chemicals, smog, and the list goes on and on. Start now; learn about the safety of your environment and food sources. Check with your local health-food store.

FATHERS-TO-BE . . . AVOID DRUGS AS WELL

Fathers-to-be should try to abstain from all drugs for up to two years prior to conception and also avoid any drug use during pregnancy that will affect the mother or baby. We do not want mothers in labor accepting drugs of any kind unless they have a complication wherein the risk of the medication is less than the risk of the complication—and such a situation should be discussed with your medical team and is rare indeed!

The American Academy of Husband-Coached Childbirth (www.bradleybirth.com; Box 5224, Sherman Oaks, California 91413-5224, 1-800 4-A-BIRTH or 1-818-788-6662), the organization that certifies Bradley Method teachers, strives for over 90 percent totally unmedicated births. The AAHCC's computer, analyzing follow-up forms received by the Academy, showed that 87.7 percent of vaginal Bradley births were completely unmedicated. No other methods come anywhere near this goal.

I personally asked Dr. Frances Kelsey of the federal Food and Drug Administration—she is the doctor who saved many American babies from armless, legless deformities by refusing to grant permission for the use of the tranquilizer thalidomide in this country—what drug I could safely give my pregnant patients. She emphatically stated, "None!" When in doubt look up information on drugs at www.FDA.gov.

DRUG DANGER IN EARLY PREGNANCY . . . HIGHEST!

The greatest danger of most drugs affecting the fetus occurs in early pregnancy, even before the first missed menses, when the mother does not even know she is pregnant. Herbs, over-the-counter drugs, teas, vitamins, homeopathy, etc., are all types of drugs and need to be carefully looked into before use. It behooves all women who might become pregnant to avoid drugs, and the same applies to their husbands.

Most people are horribly aware of the "wham" of mothers who took the tranquilizer thalidomide in early pregnancy, but it is suspected that many other drugs cause less obvious, more subtle defects in babies, that are not as easily recognized.

PLACENTA NOT A BARRIER

For years we assumed that the placenta acted as a barrier between the baby's and the mother's circulation, protecting the baby from chemicals and drugs ingested by or injected into the mother. As Dr. Kelsey stated emphatically, the placenta is now known not to be a barrier at all, rather, "It is a bloody sieve," through which everything the mother takes goes directly to the baby. This means first and foremost that the baby may get twenty times too big a dose of the drug, if a mother weighed one hundred forty pounds, her baby seven pounds. Remember, drug dosage is usually determined by the body weight of the recipient.

SELECTIVE ONE-WAY VALVE

The placenta can also act as a one-way valve, selectively concentrating drugs in the baby. As I mentioned briefly, mothers have protection for their brains with what is called the blood-brain barrier (BBB). This is a collection of capillaries in the brain that blocks or reduces the amount of drugs and unsafe chemicals crossing over or getting into the mother's brain. It is so effective that if the mother had a brain tumor and they wanted to treat it with chemotherapy the doctors would have to trick the blood-brain barrier to get it across.

BLOOD-BRAIN BARRIER

The blood-brain barrier is immature in the fetus and baby for a long time after birth. Things that seem to be okay for the mother may be harmful for the baby. One danger that has had a lot of publicity has been alcohol. We know it is harmful to babies. The question is how much alcohol can a mother safely drink. We do not know. It has been noticed that when mothers of twins drink alcohol sometimes one twin is born with fetal alcohol syndrome and the other twin does not seem to have it. How do we know the sensitivity of your baby?

CANNED TUNA FISH

Mothers should not eat excessive amounts of canned tuna fish, says the U.S. Environmental Protection Agency, because of its mercury content.

"DRUG" ERA

The historians of the future will undoubtedly look back upon the past era and refer to it as the "drug" era. The Pharmaceutical Research and Manufacturers of America estimate that ten thousand types of drugs are being manufactured in this country. We are the pill-takingest people the earth has ever known. Sir William Osler once stated: "The desire to take medicine is perhaps the greatest feature which distinguishes man from animals." Our fervent plea as advocates of natural childbirth is to imitate the animals in more ways than the physical conduct of labor; we should emulate them also in not wanting to take drugs. Due to new research demonstrating the ill effects of drugs, I hereby predict the next era, which we are on the threshold of now, will be the "drugless" era.

Prior to awareness of natural childbirth, pregnant women were taking an average of ten or more different drugs without giving a second thought to what effect this was having on the babies in their uteri. Today we have an entire new specialty in medicine, doctors who devote their time to studying babies before they are born and at birth; they are called "neonatologists." The results of their research give our great principles of unmedicated natural childbirth scientific justification.

When considering the ill effect of any chemical or drug upon the unborn child, there are several ways this "wham" may occur. The most obvious is the direct pharmaceutical effect of the drug itself. Most of the volatile anesthetics, many narcotic analgesics, and the different types of barbiturates act in this manner. In addition to the direct effect, the drug may affect the fetus by way of a metabolite or chemical change, formed either in the mother, in the placenta, or in the fetus itself. A third way the drug may affect the fetus is for it to alter the physiology of the mother to such an extent that it compromises the intrauterine environment of the baby.

"LOCAL" . . . NOT JUST LOCALIZED

A great source of irritation to me is the misnomer of a "local" anesthetic. There is no such thing! Let me use the example of a bewildered little boy taken to the doctor to have his sore throat treated. The treatment consists of being stuck with a needle in his bottom. He protests, "It's my throat that hurts, why do you treat my bottom?"

The treatment is effective because any drug, including an antibiotic, injected anywhere in the human body is rapidly dispersed from that "local" point throughout the entire body. Scalp-vein specimens taken from the unborn child have shown that so-called local anesthetic drugs placed in the mother's intrathecal area, epidural space, caudal canal, spinal canal, paracervical area, pudendal area—it matters not where—enter the baby's bloodstream within seconds after their administration.

ALL DRUGS CAN CROSS THE PLACENTA

Today some women are told that the modern drugs, such as Demerol (meperidine), Stadol (butorphanol), or the cocaine-like narcotic agents used in epidurals do not cross the placenta and cannot reach the baby. This has been proven over and over again to be untrue. Just check the *PDR*, the *Physicians' Desk Reference* (Medical Economics, 54th edition, p. 636) under Xylocaine or lidocaine; one of the most commonly used epidural agents: "*Labor and Delivery: Local anesthetics rapidly cross the placenta and when used for epidural, paracervical, pudendal or caudal block anesthesia, can cause varying degrees of maternal, fetal and neonatal toxicity.*" Check www.fda.gov for *lidocaine* and *epidural* and read what they have to say.

EFFECTS

Other effects reported have been immediate slowing and irregularity of the fetal heartbeat visible on the electronic fetal monitor, or EFM, recording, decreased newborn sucking behavior, increased incidence of jaundice, reduced uterine efficiency, drop in mother's blood pressure, a rise in the risk to the baby of adult drug addiction, a rise in the risk to the baby of an increased incidence of teenage suicide, prolonged labor, increased need for labor augmentation, additional need for forceps or vacuum extractors and cesarean sections, diminished muscle strength and tone for the first day or two of life, problems with breathing and temperature, and on and on (Doris B. Haire, "Obstetric Drugs: Their Effects on Mother and Infant," *The Encyclopedia of Childbearing*, 1992, www.aimsusa.org).

What are the long-term results? We don't know. Only time will tell, and enough time has not yet passed. What we don't know is possibly more frightening than what we do.

MEDICATED VS UNMEDICATED MOMS

When unmedicated natural childbirth was first introduced in a Canadian hospital, many years ago, I was amused to find a box of badges located in the newborn nursery. When a new shift of nurses took over, one would take the box, walk down the row of cribs, look at each baby, and then pin one of the badges on the appropriate crib. The badge asked the question, "Does your mother know you're out?"

The observant nurses had noted the difference in appearance between an unmedicated mother's baby and one whose mother had been drugged to insensibility and truly did not know whether her baby was in or out. It was obvious which were the natural-childbirth babies. They were pink, alert, anxious to breast-feed, scooting themselves up to the breast, and responsive to stimulation. They coughed or sneezed to clear their throats should mucus occlude them and, let me assure you, their mothers knew they were out.

DRUGGED BABIES ARE DIFFERENT

In contrast, the drugged mothers' babies were dusky blue, unresponsive, not interested in breast-feeding, listless, and needed to be aspirated or sucked out if mucus accumulated, because their muscles were too weak from the mothers' drugs to allow them to cough or clear their own throats. Many hospitals have a respiratory therapy team at the delivery where they try to get tubes down the baby's throat before it takes its first breath to help it breathe because of the effects of the epidural.

One of our new teachers, who works as a nursing supervisor, told me that she, too, could see which babies in the nursery had been born by natural childbirth and which had not when she came on duty.

An interesting video, *Delivery Self-Attachment*, with Dr. Lennart Righard, is distributed by Kittie Frantz, C.P.N.P. (certified pediatric nurse practitioner), a lactation consultant in California. The DVD is available from www.geddesproduction.com. It shows undrugged babies capable of scooting up to their own mother's breast after birth. Medicated babies seem to be unable to do this.

Audiometric technicians were added to nurseries in our area to test the babies' hearing by directing an electric horn at them. The horn makes an irritating noise, somewhat similar to the screeching sound produced by scraping chalk on a blackboard. If the baby was deaf, it would not respond; if it could hear, it would jump or react. When these technicians themselves became pregnant, we had a new group of young mothers coming in for unmedicated natural childbirth, for they had intelligently noticed the immediate reaction of natural-childbirth babies to this irritating sound in contrast to the sluggish, weak, delayed reaction of a baby from a drugged mother.

As an M.D. I blush with shame that what the R.N.s observed immediately took many years for doctors to notice and finally get around to studying. Research has scientifically verified the assumption I made so many years ago that drugs taken by mothers have a deleterious effect on babies.

IMMEDIATE EFFECTS OF DRUGS

What the smart nurses noted as the immediate effects of drugs—dusky color, poor muscle tone, delayed startle reaction time, inability to clear mucus, and so forth—could be compared to the small visible portion of an iceberg floating in the water, representing only the superficial visible effect. Continuing research by neonatologists, child psychologists, and the Association for Pre- & Perinatal Psychology and Health (APPPAH) (www.birthpsy-chology.com), and the interdisciplinary cooperation between the fields of obstetrics and pediatrics have extended the study of drug effects on the baby from immediate effects to behavioral long-term effects throughout the child's life.

Although it remains to be proven, we suspect mother medica-tion to produce awkwardness instead of gracefulness in the baby's later life, shortened attention span and memory ability, inability to handle stress, impaired reading ability, hyperactivity, and probably many other subtle effects yet to be discovered.

The American public is peculiarly sensitive to mentally re-tarded or crippled children—after they are delivered. Even an amateur promoter can make a fortune in donations with a cam-paign featuring pitiful pictures of crippled or retarded children. Public guilt will cause donations of thousands of dollars to their tender care. It is hard to find money that has been donated to groups advocating and teaching the prevention of these defects through childbirth and prenatal education stressing undrugged pregnancies, unanesthetized births, and normal labors brought about by training the mother and the father.

I would rather they gave pictures to the public as described in the article, "Infant Outcome in Obstetric Anesthesia" (*ICEA News* [November–December 1970]), by Dr. T. Berry Brazelton, the distinguished clinical professor emeritus of pediatrics at Harvard University: "Watching a drugged mother and a de-pressed infant who must make a 'go' with each other should stimulate us to reevaluate the routine use of pre-medication and anesthesia in pregnancy and delivery in the light of its effects on early mother-infant interaction as well as its lasting effect on their lives together."

There are many encouraging evidences of scientific and med-ical awakening to the ill effects of drugs. I attended a sympo-sium, "Drugs and the Unborn Child," sponsored by the March of Dimes and presented by Cornell University Medical College, that resulted in many new titles appearing in medical reports, such as "Expert Scores High Drug Use in Pregnancy," "Pregnant

Women Said to Take Too Many Drugs," and so forth. Where were they all, years and years ago, when I needed them? How many more babies' brains are going to be deleteriously affected before true natural-childbirth training is given to pregnant women and their husbands, enabling prevention rather than treatment of defects?

RESEARCH

Keep your eye on the continued new research in the field of long-term effects. I predict unmedicated pregnancies and births will gain the importance they have deserved, lo these many years.

New research brings new impetus and new justification for bringing babies into the world in an ideal state: babies who are breast-fed immediately and unhandicapped by the ill effects of drugs. It is a basic human right to be so born. What better endowment could we give a child?

The local newspaper printed an article and picture of one of our natural-childbirth babies: Greg Kerwin. Then thirteen years old, Greg had won a spelling contest. I feel keen memory is related to his unmedicated birth, coached by his father, Tom Kerwin, and to his being breast-fed immediately by his mother, Mary Anne Kerwin, who is one of the founders of La Leche League International. Another one of our Bradley babies, Stephanie Baldwin, became a Miss California. Her mother, Kathi Baldwin, AAHCC, is a Bradley teacher.

There are, of course, some instances where drugs and medications must be used as lifesavers for mothers. Make sure your doctor or dentist knows you are pregnant, especially if you are in the early months and your pregnancy is not apparent, for the fetus is the most vulnerable then. Discuss any use of drugs before you take them with your obstetrician/midwife, pediatrician, and pharmacist. I am pleased at the amount of information you can get from a pharmacist who has knowledge about drugs and their use and effects these days and your pediatrician is the one concerned with your baby after it is born.

Your OB or midwife focuses on the mother and baby only through the birth. There is no drug without possible side effects. Weigh the risk and benefit of anything you might take. You and your doctor need to choose the antibiotic or drug that is the safest for you and your baby.

If you have a virus infection, common cold, or flu, use immediately what I like to term "grandma" treatment—lots of liquids, fruit juice, hot soup, warm baths, steam vaporizers, hot saltwater gargles, extra covers, and bed rest. Then, if the symptoms persist, consult your doctor. At this time, no drug known is effective for viruses. Most viral infections will clear up from perspiration and bed rest. Should secondary bacterial infections occur, your doctor can take cultures and determine which antibiotic is appropriate rather than using broad-spectrum antibiotics that may contain teratogens—agents that produce physical defects in developing embryos.

WHAM TWO: INTERFERENCE WITH SUCCESSFUL BREAST-FEEDING DUE TO INITIAL SEPARATION OF MOTHER AND BABY

There are many benefits to the joyful act of unmedicated, natural childbirth, but the one that is the most outstanding to me is the privilege of the mother's handling and breast-feeding her baby immediately at its birth. In the olden days of routine drugging of women, a drug-drunken mother could not care less, and even if she wished, could not be trusted to handle her baby and manipulate it to her breast until she "sobered up" from the effects of drugs and anesthetics.

Therefore babies were necessarily separated from their mothers and cared for initially by others who usually offered the babies not the natural nipple for oral gratification but rubber substitutes filled with sugar water. Imagine the confusion of the baby later, after the mother had recovered from her drug hangover, and he was offered the mother's nipple, which was so different from the rubber one. Today, mothers may be more awake, but babies may still be affected, for example, the sucking reflex may be suppressed by modern-day drugs.

When I started, I noticed that our clearheaded, undrugged mothers, who were not strapped down or restrained in any way, eagerly, with motherly murmurs of joy, reached out to grasp and hold their babies as I placed them on their abdomens. Why not let them hold their babies? I have heard many absurd objections over the years. "The mother's hands and breasts are not sterile!" I personally feel that non-sterility is one of the greatest benefits of breast-feeding. Bacteria are essential to the alimentary canal for digestion to occur. Baby mice fed sterile milk in an absolutely sterile environment died.

Could it be that common antigens from saprophytic (harmless) skin bacteria shared by pathogenic (harmful) bacteria produce a cross-immunity that accounts for the fact that breast-fed babies are less prone to infections for the rest of their lives?

KEEPING NEWBORNS WARM . . . NATURALLY!

Another tiresome objection is that the baby will get cold unless it is put into a "warmer." A drugged baby's metabolism is reduced, and it needs all the help it can get, including heat, but a normal-term natural-childbirth baby gets all the warmth it needs from skin-to-skin contact with the mother. We instruct our circulating nurses not to wrap up unmedicated babies but to allow the mother's body to contact the baby's skin directly and then to put the warm receiving blanket over the baby and mother. You just can't get a more warm and cozy arrangement. Babies kept warm by this method generally do not need to have little beanies or booties, those little hats can be used to cover up injuries. Nature knows best: the sudden chill at birth, coming from a 98.6-degree uterus to a 70-degree room, serves the purpose of stimulating expansion of the baby's lungs. Don't we all gasp and inhale deeply when stepping out of a hot shower into a cold room? As in all animals with breasts, the next step following birth is the warm contact with mother. The immediate contentment of the baby is evidenced by the cessation of crying when put to the mother's breast. I wonder if there aren't long-term effects, too? Time and research will eventually verify this, I'm sure.

WHAM THREE: INTERFERENCE WITH SUCCESSFUL BREAST-FEEDING DUE TO POOR SUCKING REFLEX

Every species of mammal, including the human, gives birth to babies with instinctual sucking reflexes. The human baby if unmedicated will scoot to the breast and latch on and start nursing when it is ready to. Some babies nurse immediately and others take a little time. Drugged babies, if put on the mother's abdomen, show little or no interest in scooting up to the breast.

Medicated babies may have a dry mouth, which can interfere with latching on to the breast. When humans have a dry mouth they moisten their mouth with a sip of fluid before putting food into their mouth. This dryness is because of the drugs given to dry up the mother's stomach to prevent vomiting. This plus lack of sucking can interfere with the production of milk.

In contrast, natural-childbirth babies can suck vigorously. Mothers should know how to position and help them latch on correctly, as they are instructed in Bradley classes and in La Leche League meetings (www.lalecheleague.org). Incorrect positioning can cause sore nipples.

Another measurement of brain function that illustrates the ill effect of medication given to the mother in labor, is patterns of newborns' sucking, which are recorded on a pressure graph. These patterns are as individual as fingerprints.

WHAM FOUR: EFFECT ON THE BABY OF BEING SEPARATED FROM MOM

THE NEWBORN NURSERY

I'm sure the Humane Society would and should arrest me if I did to animal mothers what we do to human mothers—take their babies away from them at birth and put the babies in a big box with a glass window where the mothers could see their babies but couldn't hold them or touch them. This is not only cruel to the mothers, but what effect does it have on the babies?

Natural-childbirth babies should stay with their mothers where they can be held, loved, and breast-fed. More and more babies are put in NICU and although there is a move on to encourage parents to take more care of their infants, it is not generally continual care. Kangaroo care where the mother and baby are skin to skin makes a lot of sense and is very successful even when used with sick babies in NICU. The bonding is important for mother and baby and family.

I realize that we cannot make direct comparisons with animals, but could it be that the human effect is somewhat like that of the effects on baby rhesus monkeys in one study? The monkeys were isolated from their mothers deliberately in the revealing studies of Dr. Harry F. Harlow's work with surrogate mothers, referred to in the coming chapter on breast-feeding. These poor little cowering and mentally retarded baby monkeys are heartbreaking.

I realize human babies are of higher order, and the substitute mothers (nurses) do pick them up occasionally, but is that enough? When I first started practicing medicine, most out-of-wedlock mothers who were going to allow their babies to be adopted were delivered under anesthetic and their babies taken away. The mothers were moved to the surgical wards so as not to even see their babies. The babies were given nursery care until the adoption rigmarole was completed—interviews, paperwork, and so forth.

The length of time it took before the baby was put into the adoptive mother's arms was directly related to lowered IQ, depression, problems with memory, inability to meet stress, lowered attention span, and so on. Now we know enough to do all this paperwork first and get the baby out of the nursery, into the adoptive mother's arms, as rapidly as possible—for the sake of the baby.

The old-timers say, "A little nursery care won't hurt anything—give the mother a rest!" Psychologist Dr. Lee Salk capably demonstrated that giving just one aspect of the mother to the "inmates" of the nursery—the sound of a mother's heartbeat—made a difference in crying, in colic, in assimilation of food, in rate of growth, etc. He divided the nursery into two parts and projected the sound of a mother's heartbeat over a speaker system into one part of the nursery as referred to in the chapter on breast-feeding.

I wonder what the effects are of giving the newborn all aspects of the mother. How about not just hearing, but smelling the familiar fragrance of the mother? Of seeing her? Of tasting her? Of feeling her? Have such effects, especially long-lasting effects, been adequately studied? I don't think so! How important is initial sensory imprinting of newborns? Does the atmosphere of a hospital newborn nursery give good mental and emotional imprints?

It is interesting to note that anthropologists say that the human gestation period would be eighteen months if our babies were at the same development as other mammals. The reason humans are born at nine months is the size of the brain. Much after that they would be too big to come out. They suggest marsupial mothering like we see in kangaroos for the first nine months outside the womb.

DRUGGED MOMS NEED TO WAIT TO CARE FOR THEIR NEW BABY

If a mother has had drugs, she must wait until their effects wear off before assuming the care of her baby; this is obvious. However, our mothers who, because of complications, have anesthetics and other drugs, are encouraged to use rooming-in arrangements and keep their babies with them. The others (and with prenatal education in true natural childbirth this is around 90 percent) simply keep their babies with them and take their babies home as early as possible.

If they have had their baby in a hospital they should consider waiting at least two hours after birth as the contracting of the uterus needs to be observed that long; if the mother has missed out on a night's sleep, it might be nice to wait until the next morning to take her baby home, although some of my patients argue that they prefer to sleep at home, that a hospital is a poor place to get rest because of the unfamiliar beds, sounds, and the infernal early awakening.

"ROOM-IN" WITH MOM

We make a plea to pediatricians: let the mother "room-in" with her baby at home, by early discharging—if she had no drugs, breast-feeds, and has help at home. Pediatricians who have the reputation for doing this will have a booming practice and be sought out by modern, aware mothers. Those who persist in keeping kids in the nursery for the doctor's convenience in making rounds will be boycotted.

WHAM FIVE: EFFECT ON THE MOTHER WHOSE BABY IS SEPARATED FROM HER IN THE NURSERY

In considering the behavior of other mammals and comparing it, even indirectly, with human behavior, what is the effect on the mothers of separating babies from them at birth? Any fellow "country farmer" knows the answer to this question if he has ever taken an animal baby away then tried to return it later. If the interval of separation is very long, he can't give it back! The mother will act most unmotherly and totally reject the baby, even attack and kill it.

Human mothers, being blessed with a thick cortex to their brains, reason that the kid must be theirs—after all, it is labeled such, unless the nurses made a mistake (and many voice this fear!), so they suppose they'll have to take it! They don't totally reject the infant as the lower animals do, but do they possibly partially reject the "little stranger"? This very term implies "knock 'em out, drag 'em out" obstetrics to me.

BONDING IS ESSENTIAL (NO SEPARATION OF BABY AND MOM)

How could a mother ever consider her own baby a stranger or have the slightest doubt that this baby was hers if she was un- drugged and aware when she gave birth to it? Our marvelous mothers could pick their baby out of any crowd and never have doubts or fears of a mix-up of babies and parents. This is another blessing of our method! I remember a baby with flaming red hair—and none in either family—where both parents swore if they hadn't seen it at birth they would have claimed a mix-up of babies.

The answer to the question, "Do human mothers partially re- ject the role of motherhood if they have not had adequate con- tact with their newborns?" is a resounding, "Yes, they do." In OB/GYN News, (July 1, 1971, volume 6, number 13), an article entitled "Extended Neonate Contact Makes for Better Mother" describes the study by Dr. Marshall Klaus. The article states: "Major alterations of maternal behavior might result from per- mitting the mother of a healthy term infant to have extensive close contact with her infant in the early hours and days of life."

The mothers who were with their babies were more respon- sive to their infants' needs, more reluctant to leave them in the care of another, and more attentive during the doctor's examina- tion of the child. The article concludes: "The findings suggest that there may be a 'sensitive period' in human mothers follow- ing childbirth similar to that reported in animals." Similar con- clusions were arrived at long ago by the author of the foreword to this book, Dr. Ashley Montagu, as described in his book Touching: The Human Significance of the Skin (Columbia

University Press). This skin-to-skin contact with the baby applies in the same fashion to connect with the infant's father.

I think the time has come to design hospitals with rooming-in arrangements for the mothers with complications, and encourage mothers of natural, unmedicated births to keep their babies with them and do their "rooming-in" in their own homes.

WHAM SIX: PROLONGATION OF LABOR

One of the nicest (for the baby and parents) effects of unmedicated husband-coached natural childbirth is the phenomenal shortness of labor. Some doctors are irritated by this, as they simply can't get there in time to "catch" the baby so expertly "pitched" and feel the parents might hesitate in paying the doctor's fee. This is not true. Our parents are aware that the doctor is necessary only when the baby won't come—not when it is born so readily—and we repeatedly reassure doctors that the lifeguard gets his salary even when no lives need to be saved.

FEAR CREATED FROM THE UNKNOWN, CAUSING TENSION, LEADING TO PAIN

Untrained, unprepared mothers tend to be tense and frightened, which interferes with progress in labor. They are playing internal "tug-of-war" with their own uterus and delay the action. Other mothers, from fear, excitement, or erroneous training, tend to overbreathe or hyperventilate. This unnatural form of breathing results in abnormal loss of CO_2, tetanic contractions of the hands, and long drawn-out labors due to interference with the physiology of the uterine muscle. Drugs common today such as epidurals can also prolong labor.

WITHOUT DRUGS, AND WITH PREPAREDNESS, NATURE IS EFFICIENT

In the absence of drugs and the presence of preparedness, nature is efficient. If a mother in the first stage of labor is unable to relax, and there always are a few, we must resort to drug relaxation. The problem is that we not only relax the mother, but also the uterus—and of course the baby. Ideally, we want the mother to relax when the uterus contracts in order to obtain dilatation of the cervix. Weakening of the contractions of the uterus means a longer period of time necessary to get the job done.

NOT IN A HURRY, LET NATURE TAKE ITS COURSE!

We repeatedly tell patients we are not in a hurry; there are no trains to catch and we don't care when the baby comes, only how! A doctor who is in a hurry does not belong in the field of obstetrics. As my chief repeatedly pointed out, "An obstetrician should have a big rear end and the good sense to sit calmly thereupon and let nature take its course." We never started out to have babies sooner—it just works out that way when you don't fool around with Mother Nature.

We urge husbands as coaches to do their best to encourage these mothers-to-be to follow the simple instructions we will teach you in this book—it's a quicker, safer, and therefore better way to have a baby.

WHAM SEVEN: MATERNAL RISKS

There are human mothers still dying from childbirth even in our enlightened, medically advanced society. The medical journal *Obstetrics & Gynecology* in December 2005, reported the United States was in thirtieth place in the world. In September 2006, the same journal reported moms who choose elective cesarean ". . . have a threefold higher risk of mortality than those who choose vaginal delivery." But in my many trips through the woods in my childhood, I never ran across any dead mothers of lower animals.

NATURAL CHILDBIRTH . . . BEST FOR BIRTHING!

Natural childbirth is not only the shortest, happiest, and cheapest way to have a baby, but it is also the safest. My personal experience covering forty-six years and over twenty-three thousand babies is a zero maternal mortality rate. This is in spite of the fact that we had a high concentration of high-risk patients—kyphotic dwarfs, pneumonectomy patients, cardiac surgery patients, diabetic patients, and even the Jehovah's Witnesses who came to us in droves.

The latter are risky, of course, as their religious beliefs prevent the use of the most common treatment of the main cause of maternal deaths—hemorrhage. They will not accept blood transfusions. In spite of all this, we have never lost a mother. The immediate breast-feeding, spontaneous passage of the placenta, and good uterine contractions stimulated by breast-feeding, play an important role in preventing bleeding problems, so we welcome these patients and respect their beliefs.

HEART PATIENT STORY

I remember vividly a young couple who came into the office and wanted to know if we would accept them for natural childbirth if she got pregnant. The young wife had had open heart surgery, with a defective heart function persisting. She turned cyanotic, or blue, just from walking up the half story of steps to the office. I gently tried to talk her out of the idea, stressing the risk. She stated that she knew she couldn't live long but that she dearly loved her husband and wanted to leave him something to remember her by, and what could be better than her child? After seeing the mutual love in their eyes and the earnestness of their desires, I concurred.

They had three children with us and were most cooperative in all respects—no drugs, no anesthetics, just babies. The mother is not with us anymore—she died from an anesthetic-produced heart attack. The anesthesia was necessary due to a gallbladder attack. Her grateful husband has three beautiful children in her memory. Having a baby can be and was intended to be a natural, normal function of a woman's body. But birthing, like swimming, although a normal function, requires knowledge and training to perform. Both can be an exhilarating experience when properly performed and a very dangerous experience when fear or ignorance interferes.

Let me assure you, there is no safer way of conduct than what this book teaches. Not only are there fewer complications, but when complications do occur they can be more adequately handled due to the absence of drug toxicity and shock effect on the mother.

WHAM EIGHT: UNJOYFULNESS—"BABIES MAKE ME SICK!"

The joy of natural childbirth was illustrated by a young doctor when he was a senior medical student assigned to our hospital as an extern on obstetrics. His attention was drawn to our method when he was walking by a delivery room and heard, to his amazement, the lusty first cry of a baby, followed immediately by peals of laughter from the mother and attendants. His medical training, up to that point, had associated screams of terror and pain, not peals of laughter, with the birth of a baby. He stuck his head in the door to find out what was going on and became hooked for life on natural childbirth.

The father had rather protuberant ears; the mother had taken a quick look at the baby she had just pushed into my hands, turned to her husband, and mischievously announced to all in attendance, "Good heavens! It's got ears like the old man's, put it back!" She was laughing uproariously at her joke. Everyone present, including her husband, was laughing with her. It was a joyous, happy, true birthday party where the guests were sharing the elation of their hosts.

CHILDBIRTH FOR THE JOY OF IT

The American Academy of Husband-Coached Childbirth has a video appropriately named *Childbirth for the Joy of It*, showing the moment of birth of several couples and the ecstasy and joy manifested by both parents. I feel the most outstanding contribution of the husband is his sense of humor, and many a birth has left me with sore abdominal muscles from laughing so much at the antics of the happy parents. How different it was in the "knock 'em out, drag 'em out" era of yesterday. The medicated mothers vomited, something rarely seen in our method, only occasionally when the mother has eaten a huge meal just before labor. The mothers were actually sick from medication, but, from association, the mother's attitude toward the baby, subconsciously or even consciously, was "You make me sick."

IMPORTANCE OF FATHERS

Fathers contribute a sense of humor as well as peace and confidence to the atmosphere of a birth room, which is so very different from the delivery-room scenes of yesterday's obstetrics. As more and more parents learn to "give birth" in unmedicated childbirth, the true happiness of the birth day becomes apparent, especially when contrasted to the repulsive drug-drunken scenes of a delivery day. Think of your family's and your child's future by committing yourselves to The Bradley Method. This is one of the most rewarding investments you can make in your lives. May more and more children and families celebrate true, joyful, natural birth days and anniversaries of them rather than depressive, drugged delivery days.

How do you achieve this joyful birthing experience for you and your wife? By both of you knowing what you're doing when the time comes and being adequately prepared so you can perform as a team. Study the rest of this book carefully, do your homework as assigned, and do it well. A joyful experience bearing a child will deepen the bonds of matrimony and place a welcome sign before your child for life. It is so nice not to fool Mother Nature!

4

WHERE DO FATHERS FIT IN?

"Father of Fathers" is what couples have called me internationally. Back in 1947, I was the first doctor ever to advocate the continual presence of the father in labor and birth. It is a chuckle to see several Johnny-come-lately methods with their claims that this practice originated with them.

AMERICAN ACADEMY OF HUSBAND-COACHED CHILDBIRTH

Now in the twenty-first century, after cofounding the American Academy of Husband-Coached Childbirth, teaching Bradley classes and teacher trainings for over forty years, producing over fifty birth videos, and having six children with his wife, Marjie, Jay Hathaway is carrying on the cause of the "Father of Fathers" to future generations.

INTEGRAL PART

What do men/husbands, fathers/coaches have to do with all this? It's rather obvious that men are an integral part of making a baby. Is that all they have to do?

Frankly, when I first timidly tried out the method, I never gave the fathers a second thought. After all, my first experimental patients were young women pregnant out of wedlock, in a confinement home. I was assigned this home as part of my obstetrical training at the university. Because it was distant from the main campus and my chief put me in complete charge, I decided to apply these principles of training and preparation and see for myself what the results would be.

The patients took to the classes like ducks to water. This was possibly related to the fact that by far the majority of them were above average intelligence (and some quite brilliant academically) and also they were extremely bored. Their confinement began when their pregnant abdomens began to show, and although the administrators of the home did a fine job, the hours would drag. They welcomed with eagerness the chance to learn more about themselves and the labor to come.

Careful indoctrination was carried out, teaching the subjective feelings of labor, explanations of anatomy, stages of labor, and so on. They were then taught the objective actions of animals in these stages of labor and how they should imitate them carefully when their turns came. (For details of conduct of labor, see subsequent chapters.) To make the story more brief, they never missed any classes; they were ideal and cooperative in labor. Even though they were not going to keep their babies, they obviously enjoyed having them. The idea of "taking medicine" as part of labor and birth did not occur to these healthy young women.

Being young, and therefore naive, I enthusiastically proposed a planned control study in the main clinic at the university. I was thoroughly squelched by my superiors and laughed at by my colleagues. All well and good for OWs (out-of-wedlocks), who are noted for cooperating so well with their doctors. Just don't try it on married women with a husband to put on a show of martyrdom for. It won't work!

HUSBANDS

Husbands! I hadn't thought about them—mainly because there weren't any. I started thinking and fretting. Why should a woman, if she loved her husband and he loved her, put on a show of uncooperative martyrdom? Why were OWs so much better patients, by medical reputation, than married women? It didn't make sense. I reasoned that the OWs had a more cooperative interpersonal relationship with the doctors for the simple unflattering reason that they didn't have anyone else to whom to relate.

However, if they were married and had an ever-loving husband, that doctor would be a relatively unimportant figure. But what if they truly loved their husbands, who weren't there when their reassuring presence was needed? Then they would have to accept that poor substitute who was there, the doctor.

My head was in a whirl. Did just being married make a woman a poor obstetrical patient? Again, it didn't make sense. Being a clinician by intent, I decided the only way to find out was to see. Accordingly I asked for volunteers in natural-childbirth experiments from the world's second-most-impossible obstetrical patients—married pregnant nurses. The world's most impossible patients would be married pregnant doctors. The latter category were rare birds; there weren't enough available, although I succeeded in finding a few.

VOLUNTEERS

In the former category I was swamped with volunteers. Before I leave the wrong impression on the reader, the reason medically trained personnel (R.N.s and M.D.s) are emotionally poor-risk patients is simply that they know too much. They have seen and heard medicated maniacs in labor. They have witnessed forceps-bruised babies. Everything of a negative nature has been seared indelibly on their subconscious minds, to come back and haunt them later when they are pregnant.

As a teacher and dispeller of fear and anxiety, I get no particular sense of personal accomplishment in preparing a country woman for the birth of her baby, a woman (like the sheep rancher) whose only association with the birth process has been the peaceful, joyful births of animals she has witnessed on the farm. There really isn't much for the doctor to do. But give me a woman whose soul has been seared with negativity, and when she gives birth, after preparing with The Bradley Method, with joy and peace and without even associating medication with the act, then I feel a sense of accomplishment.

MARRIED R.N.S

Accordingly, I took the volunteer married R.N.s. Why did they volunteer? I think an article written in the local paper by an R.N. mother gives the reason in the very title: "Better Start for Babies." They had observed, as assistants, the color, muscle tone, and immediate cry of a lusty, healthy, natural-childbirth, unmedicated baby compared with the limp, blue baby of a medicated mother. The difference is obvious. Even today there is a difference between epidural and unmedicated babies.

So I trained and indoctrinated the married nurses—still thoughtlessly ignoring husbands, however. Results? In spite of the "handicap" of being married and being nurses, they were even more cooperative than the OWs. They were magnificent mothers. At this stage of my medical career, no husband, to my knowledge, had ever been allowed in that forbidding no-man's-land known as the delivery room, where the great white father of authority, the doctor, reigns supreme.

I myself had accepted these traditions without questioning. However, an event happened to jar me out of my intellectual conformity. With these experimental mothers at that time, I had allowed the husband in the labor room and frankly ignored him. When it was time to go to no-man's-land he was automatically sent to the waiting room for fathers, as was customary.

Looking back now, I don't see how I could have been so callous about a fellow man's feelings. At the time I was concentrating on a set pattern of testing the different aspects of the theory. I sat by the side of every experimental patient throughout the entire course of labor. I deliberately mistreated those wonderful mothers at regular intervals by carefully studying them objectively when they performed as instructed, then, for experimental purposes, coached them to do the opposite of what I had observed animals doing. I would then take notes on their objective appearance of pain, and correlate it later with a questionnaire to get their subjective evaluation. I was the coach and in constant attendance.

NON-TRAINED HUSBANDS

The husband sat in the labor room and did nothing and said nothing. I began to awaken to his importance when I noticed how much more calm and cooperative the patient was when her husband was present. If he left the room, even temporarily, the mother became anxious and tense and relaxed poorly with contractions. It had not dawned on me as yet to capitalize on this effect and turn the coaching over to him. That came later.

The husband was still thoughtlessly dismissed to the waiting room when birth became imminent. His wife was taken to the delivery room for the medical convenience of gadgets: special bed, lights, and so forth. Such paraphernalia is designed for the convenience of the attendants only—the mother could readily give birth in the labor-room bed, and some speedball mothers inadvertently demonstrated this with simple dexterity.

In those days, anytime an experimental natural-childbirth-trained mother was in labor the word spread around the hospital with lightning speed. As this was a teaching hospital—both student nurses and medical students—there soon came to be quite a gathering of visitors: nurses, scrub ladies, students, interns, and residents (this is in order of their importance!).

One of these nurse volunteer patients was a very attractive woman. I had sat beside her and coached her throughout labor, and when the baby was born I slipped off my "sterile" gloves and leaned over the table to shake her hand formally and congratulate her on her performance and thank her for her cooperation, as was my custom.

As I leaned over to grasp her hand, in her exuberant gratitude she suddenly grabbed me with both arms and kissed me soundly, exclaiming happily, "Oh, thank you, thank you for showing me how." My shoes were wet from the salt water that so liberally accompanies the baby's arrival, and I lost my balance and fell awkwardly against my patient, to the hilarious amusement of the onlookers. It was soon the talk of the hospital and the source of many good-natured jibes about my "bedside manner" with attractive patients.

Kidding I had grown used to, but I was suddenly shocked to serious thought as I walked back from this joyful scene to the waiting room and saw the frightened, anxious, distraught face of the man whose love and affection had been shared with this woman to produce this child.

It struck me like a sledgehammer. What on earth was this lovely woman kissing me for? Why was I the object of her gratitude as a labor coach while her young lover sat uselessly in the waiting room, fearful and anxious over his sweetheart's safety, eagerly wishing to see the outcome of his love for her, the baby, yet deprived by isolation from the most meaningful emotional experience of their lives together?

The more I thought about it, the more ridiculous it seemed. The old adage that all pregnant women fall in love with their obstetricians came to my mind; of course they may, since their husbands are not allowed to be there to share with their wives this rich emotional experience of their lives together.

Why shouldn't fathers be there? Why couldn't the role of labor coach, which as I had performed it this night had created such exuberant gratitude in the mind and soul of this mother, be performed by the baby's father? Was my ego in such a sad plight that it had to be constantly bolstered by pushing aside a real lover and accepting substitute favors from my patients? I felt more embarrassed the more I thought about it. I am not the least bit interested in having my patients fall in love with me, but I feel deeply the responsibility, as an obstetrician, to see that the act of bearing a child makes them fall more in love with the father of their baby.

I did not dream then that such a simple logical decision could result in such a barrage of obstacles and opposition from many sides and for many years to come.

The opposition has never originated from the many mothers or fathers, because once they were instructed in their roles they were eager and looked forward to the birth. No, the opposition came from fellow doctors, administrators, and nursing supervisors—a rather formidable array.

Doctors oriented in the principles of natural childbirth presented no opposition, quite the contrary. However, such doctors were then, and in most areas still are, in the minority. For such a radical innovation as fathers in delivery rooms we could not rely on a majority vote of the medical staff.

The hope for cooperative hospital rules lay in the acceptance of the administrator and his staff. Being in training at a university hospital where research was encouraged, I presented a program to the administrator as the trial of a new concept in obstetrics—total or psychosomatic obstetrics—adding psychological, emotional, and spiritual overtones as compared to the mechanical and purely medical aspects of childbearing.

After reassuring him of insurance coverage of fathers, pointing out that a father represented not an additional person present but a substitute for the anesthetist, and promising to supply the new labor coach with suit, cap, and mask similar to those worn by doctors, I was granted permission for the trial.

That was many, many fathers-in-delivery-rooms ago. The fears of the unknowing objectors have proved groundless. In my practice no father has fainted in the delivery room or otherwise made a nuisance of himself. On the contrary, the father has added an element of humor and joy and has become very much a member of the team. And regardless of the opposition, he is on the team to stay. Acceptance of these new concepts is slow but sure. The German physicist Max Planck has said, "A new scientific truth does not triumph by convincing its opponents and making them see the light, but rather because its opponents eventually die, and a new generation grows up that is familiar with it."

FOR LOVE . . .

One such father, decades ago now, John Quinn, a student at Humboldt State College in Arcata, California, made newspaper headlines when he chained himself to his laboring wife in order to foil the hospital ban on his presence. His explanation (after police were summoned) is a classical example of the increased awareness of the younger generation: "I love my wife. I feel it's my moral right as a husband and father to be there." This basic human right—to share childbirth with your wife—is expressed in the lyrics of the song, "The Green Leaves of Summer": "It was good to be young then, to be close to the earth; and to stand by your wife at the moment of birth."

CHAINS AND INJUNCTIONS

Other young men have brought legal action against hospital bans in order to achieve the same purpose. Chains and injunctions are things of the past now as hospital administrations are yielding to the demands of these young people to be able to share this important event in their lives.

It is about time that public-supported institutions give the taxpaying public what it wants! Institutions that deny the basic right of fathers in delivery rooms should be deprived of public funds. Let us not lose sight of the great underlying principle that is fundamental to the concept of a father as a participant in the birth process—preparation and training of both parents to achieve birth without the use of anesthetics rather than with the older medicated delivery.

I have often said I would hesitate to bring a yellow cur dog into a birthing room with a mother hooked up to machines, IVs pumping labor inducing drugs, lack of feeling from epidurals, blood ready to administer and respiratory therapist standing by ready to put tubes down the baby's throat before it takes its first breath.

This concept was well illustrated by the French movie *The Case of Dr. Laurent*, which opened on a scene in a tiny village with a man leading a horse out of his stable and taking it down the street to other quarters. A bystander asked the man why he was taking the horse away. His answer was that the horse had become ill from the day-and-night screaming of a woman in labor in a nearby house. The movie went on to show the elderly doctor administering another hypo to the distraught woman.

This situation is what prompted hospital rules separating husband and wife in labor. This was in the era of what I experienced and refer to as the "knock 'em out, drag 'em out" days that the movie portrays. These rules were reasonable then, and husbands had no business being near their wives. However, in view of the increasing number of Bradley instructors stressing the importance of active participation in labor by both the husband and wife with the mutual goal of spontaneous unmedicated birth, these husband-banning rules are obsolete.

"OBEDIENCE" CHILDBIRTH CLASSES

Confusion does arise when couples take "obedience" childbirth classes, as Doris Haire, president of the American Foundation for Maternal and Child Health, has labeled them, which teach only how to comply with rules. Neither mother nor father is taught the basic principles on how to birth or how to coach. Women often end up with medication and fathers simply observe. This gives a tarnished name to fathers in the delivery room because of the many dissatisfied experiences.

DIFFICULT FOR FATHERS, UNLESS . . .

Fathers may find being with their wives in labor difficult unless: (1) the wife has been trained how to perform in labor and has physically prepared her birth-giving muscles; and (2) the father has been prepared so that he understands how, why, and what his wife is doing, enabling him to coach, guide, and encourage her in a woman's ennobling work. He should be well acquainted in advance with her appearance in the various stages of labor. By being prepared for her objective appearance, he not only feels serene and self-confident through familiarity, but can apply his knowledge by acting as a coach to actually help her work with contractions.

INADEQUATELY TRAINED COACHES

It is cruel to encourage inadequately trained coaches to participate in this special event. She, in turn, feels secure knowing that her ever-present coach not only loves her but knows what she is about and how to guide her. As one experienced natural-childbirth mother peacefully expressed it, "As long as he's there I know he won't let me goof." And (3) the couple has practiced labor rehearsals over and over again, in class and at home.

"HUSBAND"

We do get objections to the word "husband." Our definition of a husband is someone who loves and protects this woman. It is someone she can depend on and relate to. It is generally the father of this child who wants the chance to bond to this new baby that they conceived together. Husbandry is what they teach at universities when they breed cattle, the word doesn't have to mean "married." You can "husband" your resources.

BEST FOR BIRTHING

Husband-coached childbirth is achievable for all. It is the best way to give birth and sets the standard. "Husband" or "husbandry" is the act of involvement in such a capacity as to facilitate tremendous bonding and support. One does not have to be the biological father or a Y-chromosome person to have this title. Mothers who are unwed by choice or circumstance, nontraditional families can choose a special "significant other" that they depend on and relate to in very special ways.

There is simply no other word in English that conveys the same tender bond that a coach shares and experiences. A "husband" is one who is dedicated and supportive of this woman, willing and anxious to serve and defend her like no one else can, in labor, birth, child rearing, and life. The role of "husband" is the basis of what we teach and what has made The Bradley Method so successful. Women used to labor alone. "Husbands" missed out on the amazing bonding that happens when they are present at a birth. Why is it that some men hesitate to be around birth? Some think it is "woman's work," some don't realize they are important to the process, they are afraid they might get in the way. They don't know they can help. They don't realize how significant they are.

WHOSE JOB IS IT?

1. Who will go with the mother to classes to learn what to expect and how to help her in labor?
2. Who will encourage her to exercise during pregnancy?
3. Who will encourage her to eat well every day?
4. Who will help her in early labor?
5. Who will call the doctor or midwife when she's in labor?
6. Who will sign the admitting forms and answer questions?
7. Who will keep her relaxed?
8. Who will remind her to slow her breathing and relax again after something disturbs her?

9. Who will recognize the natural alignment plateau (NAP) and keep her from getting discouraged?
10. Who will spoon ice chips into her mouth?
11. Who will wipe her sweaty brow while she is working hard?
12. Who will she rely on to keep watch and help her to avoid unnecessary pain?
13. Who will she depend on to tell her she's doing a great job over and over and over and over again?
14. Who will act as an advocate for the mother when decisions must be made?
15. Who will know what relaxes her?
16. Who will rub her sore back?
17. Who will hold her up in the shower if she wants to take one?
18. Who will sit with her in the bathroom when she wants to labor in there?
19. Who will help her find a good pushing position?
20. Who will hold her up in the pushing position, even for hours, if necessary?
21. Who will remind her to push to the point of comfort?
22. Who will relax her between contractions?
23. Who will tell her when you can see the head?
24. Who will share this special time of bonding?
25. Who will the mother say she couldn't have done it without?

The coach has a lot to do!

Do you want more jobs the husband is ideally suited for with a laboring woman? See the complete list of questions in *The Bradley Method Student Workbook*. The job is massive and amazing. As the husband you are well suited for the job.

5

PREPARATION AND FIRST-STAGE LABOR

What Do Animals Do?

Animal fathers' presence in labor may be unnecessary or unnoticed, as the animal mother can rely on her instinctive know-how and needs no coaching. The father may play a role of protector that humans do not see. Your wife, lacking this instinct and education, must be supported, loved, guided, directed, and encouraged.

When a pregnant woman does not have a husband for this role I insist that she have a coach, someone she can depend on and relate to. This could be her significant other, friend, brother, sister, mother. I do feel it is important that this person, if possible, be someone the baby will bond to at birth and grow up in a close relationship with. Since most of the time this important person is the husband, I will continue to refer to the husband. After all, in college they call the study of animal reproduction "animal husbandry."

If your wife is to handle herself in labor as other animals do, let us carefully observe their conduct to see what we can learn. Although almost any species of lower animals would serve as an example, let's take one that is domesticated, say the cat or dog, for convenience, and observe them in labor.

FIRST SIGN—RESTLESSNESS AND RETURN TO HER NEST

The first sign that an animal is in labor is restlessness. The animal will pace about, sit or lie down awhile, then restlessly get up and walk some more. In human beings I refer to the initial intermittent walking stage as the "putsy-putsy" stage, as no distinct pattern is established and the mother just "putsies" around. As the labor progresses and contractions get closer and harder, the animal mother then returns to her nest, or where she sleeps at night, for the next phase of first-stage labor, the imitation of sleep.

DO NOT LIKE TO BE OBSERVED

The next observation will be that animals do not like to be observed in this phase of labor—by anyone. They become secretive, coy, and cunningly try to make this a private party. The family cat does not perform this deed out on the sidewalk or in any obvious place. She will, if left alone, probably perform at night and retire to the same location where she sleeps. She does not want observers. There seems to be a great need to concentrate on the job at hand and the animal knows this need and resents distractions. Even a favorite dog, known for its good temper and loving nature, will snap or bite its master if disturbed in labor.

We have already gained a point in the necessity for training fathers as labor attendants. They must not do anything that will distract or disturb their wives during labor, or they may be verbally snapped at. This does not mean the laboring mother (be it dog or human) has lost her love for the master or father. Rather it points out the fundamental commandment of nature: laboring mothers should not be disturbed or distracted; they have a great need for deep concentration. If this concentration is disturbed, pain and prolongation of labor result.

RHESUS MONKEYS

At a district childbirth convention held in Madison, Wisconsin, we were privileged to take a tour through the primate laboratories where Dr. Harry F. Harlow and his associates were studying mother-child relationships in rhesus monkeys. Their work involved the study of the results of early separation of baby monkeys from their mothers at an average of seven hours from birth and subsequent exposure of the babies to surrogate or substitute mothers of varying characteristics.

I questioned the guide who was conducting the tour as to why they didn't separate the babies immediately after their birth. The answer was that for purposes of the study, that would be ideal, but that it was impossible. The mothers always gave birth at night, but when humans stayed up to separate the infant monkeys immediately, the mother's labor would become irregular and even cease because of the emotional disturbance created by the presence of the human intruder. If disturbing a mother's emotions in labor so drastically affected uterine action in rhesus monkeys, could this be true also in human mothers?

In lecturing student nurses it is stressed that the labor room should be darkened by pulling the shades in daylight. Although human mothers have apparently lost the instinctual ability to bear their young always at night, a darkened room is still of benefit. Labor rooms at night should be dimly illuminated from the sides, never by overhead lights—except if needed momentarily by the midwife, nurse, or doctor.

Now, back to the family cat or dog in labor. By quietly, even sneakily, approaching, we observe additional factors involved.

NEEDS IN LABOR

1. **The need for darkness and solitude.** Bright lights are indeed disturbing. My attempts to take photographs of dogs and cats have been foiled by the indignant laboring mothers' retreating to dark secluded places—usually

physically out of reach of annoying human beings—such as far under the house or barn.

2. The need for quiet.   This is obvious. Any loud or unexpected noise disturbs the mother. Again we make the fervent plea to attendants in hospital labor sections to keep raucous noises down to a minimum. One careless, loudmouthed person can undo months of prenatal preparation.

3. The need for physical comfort during first-stage labor.
This is made manifest by animals in many ways. On the farm we could predict the imminence of labor when the pregnant cat would be seen carefully digging out a hollow place for its body in the warm earth under the barn. It would test out the area by lying in it, then diligently paw away any lump or irregular area until its body fit the cavity in the earth without any disturbing localized pressure.

A few years ago our beloved family dog, a French poodle, was pregnant, and the children noticed with delight how several days before the birth occurred the dog dutifully raided the soiled-clothes basket in the basement, selecting articles of soft material, and laboriously dragged them up the steps to her basket in the kitchen. Here she meticulously lined the basket with them, turning around and carefully pawing away any lumps until she was satisfied with the comfortable contour. Wise mother that she was, she was upset by the attention her acts were bringing from the overly interested children and after the household was asleep, cunningly transferred her nest padding to a closet left open in the bathroom. She gave birth to her puppies peacefully and quietly during the night without arousing a soul—much to the disappointment of the children.

Observation of animals, then, points out the need for a comfortable position of the mother's body during labor. For years human mothers—and their doctors!—have been guessing wrong when labor will begin. How does the animal mother having her first pregnancy know in advance to so prepare?

I'll leave the answer to that question to the academic doctors—I can't answer it and, as yet, neither can they—but as a clinical doctor may I strongly point out that animals do know and that this observed fact is not weakened in the least by our human ignorance of how they know. The scientific eye of human learning is just now beginning to look timidly into the function of animal brains and instinctive abilities— and it has a long way to go.

4. **The need for physical relaxation.**   These itemized needs are not mutually exclusive. Relaxation even in animals takes concentration. When this concentration is disrupted (by bright lights, loud noises, uncomfortable positions, presence of strangers) the animal tenses up, and tensing up during uterine contractions produces in animals the same thing it does in human mothers in first-stage labor—pain! Again, we do not know how academically, but we jolly well do know clinically that it does.

We encourage any human mother not to "believe" a word we state on the concepts we are teaching. We respect intelligent, honest skepticism. Being a man, and therefore destined never to know the actual feelings of labor, I have always, from the first experimental patient years ago to women in labor today, challenged them to believe nothing but to try everything proposed, and then tell me if there is a difference.

I throw this challenge to the reader: carefully coach your wife in first-stage labor in the details of relaxation, then ask her to tense her voluntary muscles deliberately (any muscle—it doesn't matter which) during the next uterine contraction and then tell you the effect of such deliberate tensing. Try it and see what she says! No wonder the animal mother will try her best to avoid such disturbances and actually attack even a loved human being if he persists in disturbing her concentration!

Animal mothers are observed to lie absolutely still and physically relaxed during the contraction of their uterine muscles. Like efficient athletes, the muscles not being utilized in the event are completely inactive and relaxed, enabling the energies of the body to be more effectively directed to the one that is being utilized. My friends have laughingly said that I bore people to death by seeing manifestations of natural-childbirth principles in everything and anything.

The basketball player going in for a setup shot at the basket is graceful and lithe—the arm not being used in this one-arm shot is limp and relaxed. The football player getting set to kick the crucial placekick that may win the game is a picture of deliberate relaxation as he shakes tension from his shoulders and arms to increase the effectiveness of his leg muscles.

The mother, whether by instinct or training, who deliberately loosens her other muscles during her uterine contraction is rewarded by comfort (nature's reward for helping rather than hindering birth) and by effectively producing the desired result (shortening of time required).

5. The need for controlled breathing.   Animals breathe in first-stage labor in the same fashion as in sleep. Because labor is what the term implies—hard work—the breathing is deeper and, as labor progresses, more rapid. Here confusion arises, as some species of animals do not perspire. Body heat is increased due to the forcefulness of the uterine contractions. In animals with perspiration mechanisms, and this includes the human, cooling is achieved by perspiration.

Other animals are observed to break into panting type of breathing, at intervals, which serves as their particular mechanism to cool their body. Most animals, particularly if the environment is warm, breathe through open mouths rather than the narrower air passages of the nostrils. This may be related to the need for a greater volume of air or, as some have suggested, the relaxation of the jaw muscles as part of the overall state of generalized relaxation. This is why I based my method on the observation of perspiring mammals.

6. The need for closed eyes and the appearance of sleep.   Again this is probably only a manifestation of the need for absolute and total concentration. It results in the label of the first stage of labor as that of the "sleep" stage. Animals return to their sleep place, lie, breathe, and look as if they are asleep during first-stage labor. The irritation that they manifest at the presence of human beings may be related to their distrust and need for keeping an eye on the intruder even when the human being is inactive. This again interferes with the increased ability to concentrate that comes from shutting out visual stimuli. Closed-eye concentration seems to be a necessary aspect of their job.

WHAT SHOULD HUMAN MOTHERS DO?

The answer to this question by the hypothesis of the natural-childbirth concept is, of course, that human mothers should do the same thing!

Because of slight structural differences of the human body, and because of considerable differences in the human soul, we now need to take the animal observations we have made and apply them one by one to this complex and highly developed mixed-up animal known as the human being. What works for other animals may work for us. Let's try it.

In the video *Bradley on Birthing,* Dr. Bradley condensed the needs into a short checklist for the mother. During the "putsy-putsy" stage, or the "get ready" stage, the mother can generally walk, sleep, shower, eat, drink, etc.

MOTHER'S CHECKLIST
(Active First-Stage Performance Needs)

During active first stage, the mother's performance needs begin with sleep imitation with her eyes closed, which is reflected in these points:

1. **Do not move** . . . during a contraction. If she does it will hurt and she will lose her concentration. Between contractions she can move as she wishes.

2. **Abdominal breathing** . . . is normal for human beings. It is efficient, effective, and helps with relaxation.
3. **Relaxation** . . . is an amazing pain-management tool and the key to handling pain for a successful birthing environment. When the mother relaxes she allows the uterus to do its work. The uterus will move forward, putting the baby in the proper alignment with the pelvis, making it easier for the baby to be born.
4. **That "duh" look** . . . really means relaxing your jaw, which relaxes the rest of your body making it still easier for the baby to be born.

Animals like quiet, dark, comfortable, secluded places to give birth to their young. They do not like the presence of strangers. Well, we have a big problem right off the bat. Doctors want human mothers to have babies in hospitals, and these requirements would hardly be achieved by the environment of any hospital. They are most nearly met by the environment of a mother's bedroom in her own home and the reassuring nearness of familiar and loved faces rather than those of strangers.

As a doctor and advocate of natural childbirth I can have no arguments with Ashley Montagu and other experts on human relations who contend that from a bacteriological, sociological, psychological, moral, and spiritual standpoint, human babies should be born at home. The home environment appears to best fulfill the requirements I have itemized. However, as an obstetrician I honestly felt that babies should be born in hospitals.

Why? Because there is an irreducible incidence of complications in human obstetrics, and hospitals are best equipped for immediate management and correction of some of these complications. Hospitals also introduce new complications that home births don't have. Some complications can be foretold, but others cannot. It would be convenient to have the many uncomplicated births at home and only the complicated ones at the hospital.

Since my retirement I have observed some hospitals that actually increase the childbirth risks by their mandatory interventions.

Some couples realize they would be better off at home instead of hospitals. We must not alter the great advances already made in the medical and scientific aspects of obstetrical management, but they are useless without human consideration. Home or hospital needs to be seriously considered and decided upon after much thought.

Natural-childbirth principles add to, not detract from, the established principles of obstetrics. They should add what has been lacking, proper and complete preparation of both husband and wife for their introduction into parenthood. In my practice about 3 percent of our patients needed cesarean sections. Of the remainder who have had their babies through the vaginal route, 96.4 percent achieved spontaneous, uncomplicated, unanesthetized births that could have been properly managed at home. However, there was still that 3.6 percent who needed hospital-equipped management of sometimes unforeseeable complications.

From a medical standpoint, then, both home and hospitals present unique benefits and risks. This does not, however, alter one bit the importance of the great principles we follow. It does present the formidable task of altering the hospital environment to make it conform with the home environment as closely as possible. Since most couples choose the hospital I will assume you have made this choice. The principles in this book work anywhere you give birth—hospital, home, birth center, even unexpected situations such as in the car on the way.

Years ago when the full realization of the task of altering the hospital environment became apparent, it was almost overwhelming. Maternity hospitals were cold, gaunt, impersonal halls of barren stone cluttered with strange gleaming steel gadgets of awesome appearance, ruled over and run by eagle-eyed matrons policing a list of rules and regulations that would choke a horse. They were about as remote from a secluded home environment as one could get. Guilt-ridden husbands were glared at and told to stay in the waiting room—that chamber of horrors where nervous, distraught, useless, cigarette-smoking clowns paced the floor.

HOME ENVIRONMENT

The home environment must be reproduced as much as possible in the hospital. Many little changes—in decor, subdued noise, more human and warmer attitudes by personnel—were brought about. However, the most important factor, and the one most desired by the mothers, was the inclusion of the husband with the wife throughout labor and birth. In most localities this has been achieved.

Today, through the noble efforts of many devoted workers, family-centered childbirth, which includes having husbands at the birth, is being introduced into more and more hospitals. Have your local Bradley Method childbirth educator, certified by the American Academy of Husband-Coached Childbirth, recommend a doctor, midwife, or physician's assistant who can assist you in a supportive hospital, home birth, or birth-center situation that encourages you to share childbirth with your wife.

Now, let's get back to how you are going to help your wife imitate the lower animals in the conduct of her labor. Most family-centered maternity hospitals have a preliminary guided orientation tour for you and your wife. By all means take advantage of this tour and become familiar with the appearance of the labor and birth room. Knowing where you're going and what it looks like is important, too.

There are certain necessary nuisances you should be aware of when you enter the hospital with your wife in labor. Most hospitals have some procedures that are standard after the paperwork of admitting is completed. This may include changing into their gown, doing additional paperwork, giving urine and blood samples, running a strip on the external fetal monitor, having vital signs taken, answering questions, etc.

HUSBAND AND WIFE SHOULD *NOT* BE SEPARATED

There generally is no reason for husband and wife to be separated. If she needs you, do not leave her side. Part of being a good coach is to contact the business office of the hospital in advance during her pregnancy and find out what is required of you at the time of admission. While this varies with each hospital, make as many arrangements beforehand as possible. Ask for copies of any forms that need to be signed when you arrive so that you can read and think about them in advance without the distraction of contractions.

CHANGING CLOTHES

In the labor room some hospitals require you to remove outside clothing and may or may not have you don a father's "hatching jacket," as our husbands fondly call these coats. Wear it with pride. It is the label of a birth coach and is indeed a mark of distinction. Wear your COACH button from class and be sure the nurse sees your Bradley Coach Card signed by your instructor. Have *The Bradley Method Student Workbook* nearby, always!

MAP OF LABOR

As an overview of the map of labor (see page 66) I reminded them my practice was in colorful Colorado, and we utilized a comparison of mountain climbing to that of labor to help both husband and wife know what to expect. In the early stages of labor the uterus is not working particularly hard or particularly often. Some labors skip this part or go through it quite rapidly to the more advanced type. If your wife is still in early labor there is generally no need for her to stay in bed.

Preliminary Stage (putsy-putsy)	First Stage	Transition Stage	Second Stage

RELAXATION

Relaxation takes deep concentration and should be saved for later, more vigorous labor. We refer to this early labor as the gentle "foothills" that precede the higher mountains, or it is called the "putsy-putsy" stage. Some couples opt to stay home during this time. Others head for the hospital because of traffic, distance, or progress of labor. The uterus will contract occasionally as you stroll around with your wife. This results in a feeling of pressure in her abdomen, back, or pelvis, and she may want to stop momentarily and lean over. Husbands are good leaning posts, and during these few seconds she should bend over slightly, relax completely leaning on you, and lightly breathe through parted lips until the contraction lets up—then you may amble on your way.

There will probably be a lounge where you two may sit for a while during the foothill phase. Between contractions she will be in a conversational mood and chat with you, just as you two would were you climbing the foothills. There are occasional little steep parts where you must concentrate momentarily on the job of climbing. But there are regular declines and flat areas where again there is no particular need for concentration, and idle chatter can be resumed. You will find your wife to be her usual good conversational self during these rhythmical phases. Your very presence is an overwhelming relief from boredom to your wife. She has nothing particularly to share, conversationally, with strangers (nurses, doctors, or otherwise), but she does with you.

As time goes on, the foothills become a little steeper, the inclines are longer, and the periods necessitating concentration become longer—the declines progressively get shorter and less frequent. These declines will gradually fade out, as will her desire for carrying on conversation as the mountain gradually changes and becomes steeper. After good, firm, regular uterine contractions are established, when she wishes to go to bed, escort her back to the labor room, leisurely, for there is no hurry. The shortest labors, remember, occur in an atmosphere of peace and calmness, and your attitude and appearance can do much to promote this.

Now comes the more active part of your role as a coach. The uterine muscle is now getting down to real business, and your wife should now carefully imitate the other animals in her conduct during uterine contractions. It really doesn't matter much what she does between uterine contractions, but it matters very much now what she does during them.

Let's get back to our observations of what nonhuman animals do in labor and carefully apply them to your wife's conduct now.

LABOR NEEDS THE COACH CAN HELP WITH

We have established needs for (**Need One**) a dimly lit room where there is (**Need Two**) quiet and privacy. Pick a hospital where family-centered principles are practiced (if you need help, ask for it from your Bradley teacher).

Now let's consider (**Need Three**), the need for physical comfort, as observed in the instinctive careful preparation of the "nest" by animals. How does this apply to your wife now, in labor?

First-stage labor in animals was briefly described as sleep imitation. Although they were not asleep, they looked like it and were positioned as in sleep. It behooves you as a husband, then, to have a good idea of how your big-tummied wife positions herself at home in her own bed while asleep. During the last few months of pregnancy you should make careful observations of her position in bed, the relationship of her arms, legs, etc., when she is deeply asleep.

OBSERVE HER SLEEPING

Try not to awaken her if you come in late one night, and carefully study her while she sleeps. She then presents the identical picture we want you as a labor coach to help her assume now in the hospital, by your careful guidance during her uterine contractions. This same position that she selected at home as being the most comfortable for her should be repeated at this stage of labor.

You will notice on the flat bed at home how she does not lie flat on her back—not at three a.m. during the last months of pregnancy. Some women may consciously start out the night lying on their backs because they wrongly believe that they might hurt their baby if they lie on it. However, once their conscious mind is asleep, or partially so, they will subconsciously turn over on their sides, curl up in a ball, and adjust the pillow or pillows to the particular contours of their bodies. They usually sigh a deep, contented sigh as they achieve their particular position (this is strictly individual for every mother) and comfortably doze away.

Today we know lying on the back during pregnancy may put pressure on the blood vessels leading to the uterus and decrease the oxygen supply to the baby. This could put the baby at risk.

In the last few months some mothers like to have a second pillow to support the top leg, which is raised up higher than the bottom leg to rotate the hips, allowing the heavy uterus to fall freely away from the mother and toward the bed. Have an extra pillow available in these later months of pregnancy and suggest that your wife try out different combinations of support. Suggest, don't dictate. She will, by experience, work out her own positional pattern on her side. Having observed it, you, as husband and coach, should be very familiar with it; now, in first-stage labor, help her duplicate it in the hospital bed.

ASK FOR IT . . .

If you need an additional pillow, ask for it. If it is wintertime and your wife mentions that her feet are cold (and some do even in summer), also ask for a hot-water bottle, heated rice or corn bag/sock, or extra blanket. Make her physically comfortable. Know her little idiosyncrasies in advance. Such attentive care endears you to her and helps her to relax so her body can do what it was built to do.

Monotony and boredom constitute handicaps in the first stage of labor. This is the period when the forces of the uterine muscle must thin out and stretch the opening, called the cervix, through which the baby is to leave the uterus and enter the birth canal. This stage can be boring because the mother is required during the muscular action to simply "get out of the road" and let the action alone. This stage of do-nothingness is monotonous and takes great concentration on her part. Your very presence alone helps immensely, but there are other things you can do also.

One of these things involves an occasional change of her position. At home on her flat bed there is only the one position for relaxation; curled up on her side. This involves an infinite number of variations in arm, leg, and pillow positions, differing from one person to another—e.g., some mothers put the lower arm underneath and along their backs, others snuggle this arm under the pillow, and so forth. You should be familiar with your wife's variations from your observations at home.

In the hospital, however, there is an additional position possible that your wife may find quite comfortable and which you cannot practice at home in advance. This is due to the adjustable nature of hospital beds compared with the one at home. (I advise a husband whose wife is carrying twins or an extra-large amount of salt water—and therefore larger distension of the abdomen—that he can win further endearment by renting a hospital bed during the last month for use at home.)

ADDITIONAL POSITION

The additional position for first-stage labor involves elevating both the upper and lower part of the hospital bed so your wife can assume a lounge-chair or contour-chair sprawl. She is neither sitting up nor lying down—rather, in between these two. The two pillows are now used, folded up, under her arms and elbows to support them. Her knees should be sprawled, unladylike but mother-like, comfortably apart.

The actual degree of elevation of either the upper or lower part of the bed should be, again, individually worked out by having her tell you what she prefers—after several trials. No pillow is usually used under the head, as the head can be raised farther with the action of the bed if she wishes. Her arms and hands would otherwise fall awkwardly to her sides and interfere with relaxation unless pillows are folded to support the elbows and serve as armrests.

This position is based on the scientific principle that a group of muscles under tension cannot relax properly. All movable parts of the bone joints should be at the halfway station of the extent of their movement. Neither fully flexed (bent) nor fully extended (straightened), but rather at a happy medium of half and half. This you should consider as a coach in positioning your wife's wrists, elbows, shoulders, hips, knees, ankle joints, and so forth, as you adjust the bed and pillows.

As an illustration this point was brought to me forcibly when I was still experimenting early in my career with the group of nurses having their first babies. I was being ridiculed by some colleagues over the apparent lack of benefit of the relaxation teaching on one of our experimental patients. She was unable to achieve full relaxation and in general acted as if she had had no training at all in how to conduct herself during labor.

I had positioned her (pre-husband-participation days) in this contour- or lounge-chair position as part of the experiment. She had, up to then, been such a calm, capable person that I was bewildered at her inability to relax fully during contractions. As I could see no reason for this, I asked her what she thought was interfering. She apologized over such a seemingly trivial thing— said she felt sort of silly—but the covers were bound down too tightly at the end of the bed and they held her feet down, forcibly pointing her toes, which made it impossible to relax.

As soon as the problem was recognized and corrected by loosening the covers, she relaxed perfectly and performed magnificently for the rest of her labor. There is no detail too fine to be ignored in achieving the necessary degree of physical comfort required in labor. Don't hesitate to ask your wife for suggestions of what else you can do to make her comfortable.

Depending on the length of labor (and this is quite variable with every baby), your wife may want to alternate between this contour position and her old home one occasionally for variety. Try switching positions back and forth once in a while. Or if she prefers one position over the other and says so, fine, don't argue—only she knows how she feels. We have seen some flexible-jointed slim ladies draw one or even both feet up and, with their knees wide apart, rest their feet against the raised lower part of the bed. Since no two people are alike, we cannot dictate exactly how your wife should be positioned.

LYING ON YOUR BABY

On a flat bed she should lean on her baby, never the reverse, her baby on her. Reassure her that she cannot hurt a baby by lying on it (it's floating in salt water that equalizes any pressure), but it can jolly well hurt her by lying on her.

Never, never should your wife lie for any length of time

flat on her back with her baby on top of her. Although this is sometimes necessary for short intervals to allow medical examinations, it is not only deucedly uncomfortable but also reduces blood flow to the heart and the kidneys and should never be a position in labor.

If you're ever out in the woods and find a pregnant animal lying flat on its back, balanced on its backbone, go get a spade and come back and bury it! No living pregnant animal would mistreat itself so.

I'll never forget the sight I beheld when I scouted a hospital to see if I wanted to bring my patients there, just before starting my practice. What I saw and heard made me run in terror and look elsewhere. A nurse was applying a restraining straitjacket-like device on a laboring mother, strapping her flat on her back so she couldn't move. While adjusting the straps the nurse was complaining to the patient: "Every time I come to check you you're lying on your side. I told you to stay on your back so I can check your baby. Now we'll see if you mind," she added as she busily applied the restraining straps.

The mother was a wild-eyed medicated maniac, all conscious control long gone via drugs. She had just enough brain function left to know how much better it felt to lie on her side, and yet she was being deprived of that! In all fairness to the attending nurse, she had never been in labor herself and no one had ever informed her that a mother's position in labor makes a world of difference in how she feels. This is, I repeat, not the nurse's fault. It is rather the fault of the lack of awareness of the medical profession. Nurses follow doctors' orders.

If doubts exist in your mind whether position in labor affects how a woman feels, try it and see. You can momentarily experiment together, just as I did many years ago with volunteer nurse mothers. You have nothing to lose but much to gain. To the best of your ability, help your wife position herself as has been outlined for first-stage labor. Now ask your wife to disobey any of our positional rules during a uterine contraction—e.g., lie flat on her back or in any awkward, strained position—and see what she says. Is there a difference?

This challenge of "try it and see for yourself" we suggest after every itemized point of conduct that we have gleaned from observing animals in labor. Natural-childbirth principles are not idly arrived at by armchair philosophical theory but are based upon observed facts.

NEED FOUR

We now come to (**Need Four**) observed in animals, physical relaxation of uninvolved muscles during labor. This represents the aspect technically most difficult for human imitation. Any stressful situation human beings encounter is met with the defense mechanism of muscular tension. Prior to the recognition of the stresses of life, human babies' muscles, when not in use, are automatically perfectly relaxed.

As the stresses begin to accumulate (bowel training, personal neatness, making good grades, facing competition, keeping up with the Joneses, approaching parenthood, bossy mothers-in-law) the human being responds with tension. Inability to cope with stress is reflected in excess tension—tension headaches, spastic colons, nervous stomachs retaining gastric secretions too long due to muscular spasm until ulcers develop, and so forth. In addition to the cluttered emotional-mental state of human beings, which interferes with relaxation, there is a physical barrier to be overcome.

To perform any physical feat with grace and dexterity, the human being must practice and practice to achieve relaxation of uninvolved muscles. Such simple acts as running, jumping, even walking, are instinctively performed gracefully and automatically by nonhuman animals. Grace in physical action is a result of ability to keep the uninvolved muscles relaxed, an economy of muscular action. This does not mean we human beings cannot achieve physical feats similar to those of animals. It means, rather, that we must recognize the human need for practice and physical conditioning of our muscles in the apparent absence of human instinct.

PRACTICE IS IMPORTANT

Some people can run with the grace of a gazelle, swim like a fish, etc., but such abilities are acquired and maintained through practice.

Here, again, comes the factor of individuality. We are all different. Some humans need far more practice than others to achieve the same physical goals. This, topped by the heavy human overlay of emotional factors, creates quite a complex picture.

To the repeated inquiry, "Do you think every woman can learn to do natural childbirth?" I counter with another question. Do you think every woman, in the absence of physical abnormalities, can be taught to swim? They are both acts instinctively performed by animals. We have to contend with individual variations again. Some humans take to water like ducks, others are rigid and fearful of water. The human emotional factor is important.

An inexperienced woman who has been thrown into deep water against her wishes and nearly drowned is a very real challenge to a swimming instructor for the rest of her life. The very thought or sight of water makes her rigid with fear. Nevertheless, with calm reassurance and step-by-step training, even she can still be taught to swim. One of our teachers, Coni Sherman, AAHCC, said that natural childbirth may not be for every mother but it is for every baby.

Similarly, some women take to natural childbirth with ease and grace and a minimum of coaching. Others, especially if they have had a frightening experience in childbirth previously, take a lot more practice and more patient, reassuring coaching. Both types can reach the same success; the coaching technique is different.

The farm girl who has known only the peace and happiness of animal births is an easy coaching case (e.g., the sheep rancher cited previously). I get much more personal satisfaction out of the challenge of high-strung "nervous" patients who, when we first meet them, are scared to death to have a baby. Is there such a thing as a woman who is too nervous and high-strung to utilize natural childbirth? Good heavens, this is the type who, above all others, needs natural childbirth. I have an ego-deflating feeling that the female sheep rancher could have performed perfectly well on the range without having ever been near a doctor.

I remember reading a fascinating story by the charming actress Julie Harris on the birth of her first baby. Her doctor dismissed natural childbirth as not applicable in her case, because as an actress she was too nervous and high-strung.

She returned home in despair and tears to report this to her husband. He, however, had read up on natural childbirth and it was obvious to him that the doctor had not. The husband indignantly maintained this wasn't true and he would teach her himself! He proceeded to work with his wife at home, practicing the principles with her in careful preparation for the birth. He then accompanied her to the hospital and served as her coach. Can you think of a better coach than an attentive, educated, loving husband?

Result: She gave birth to the baby rapidly and joyfully before the doctor got there! When, during the labor, the attending nurses attempted to send the husband-coach away, Julie vehemently stated, "When he leaves, I leave." I think the attendants got the message: she meant business. He was essential to the task at hand and she knew it.

Your wife can be shown the principles of relaxation and she can be taught the consciousness of her muscles' state of tension in prenatal classes under the supervision of experienced teachers. Being a human animal, however, she needs to practice these principles at home daily in order to perfect them. This you can help her do. A suggested time is just before retiring for the night, as a prelude to sleep. This serves a double purpose: it establishes her self-confidence in her physical relaxation ability, and it is an aid to peaceful slumber.

"LETTING GO"

We have found the following step-by-step pattern of deliberate awareness of "letting go" muscle tension in definite body areas, one after the other, to be most effective. Starting from the top down, relax the forehead, eyelids, face muscles, jaw, neck, shoulders, arm muscles, chest, back, abdomen, hips, thighs, legs, and feet. This steplike progression should be accompanied with a gentle, light touch of the various areas, stroking lightly with the fingertips. The husband-coach should give verbal suggestions of relaxation in a diminishing volume of voice, ending with nearly a whisper.

Test your wife's ability by gently lifting and dropping her hand, gently shaking her foot or ankle, gently rolling her head from side to side to make her aware of any residual neck tension. Her position during this practice at home should be her individual sleep position on her side, which you have helped her arrive at by observing her during deep sleep.

Do not have her try to maintain this deep conscious relaxation for long intervals. This is practically impossible over extended periods, and, besides, the uterine muscle hardly ever contracts for more than one minute. Interrupt your practice at home with stretch sessions and low back rubs.

The baby box (in Latin called a uterus) is a heavy organ and is fastened to the mother only in the low back area by a set of muscles called the uterosacrals, going from the uterus to the sacrum or "saddle" area. This is the curved area of the lower back where, if your wife will pardon my illustration, the saddle would be placed on a horse. Rub this area firmly and slowly with the heel of your hand. Lubricate the skin with her favorite lotion to allow your hand to slide freely. She'll probably murmur approval—it feels good! These muscles get tired carrying babies around all day; massage them firmly at bedtime. Now, at an agreed signal, imagine the return of another uterine contraction, and for one minute teach her to carefully relax. Warm relaxation replaces cold tension as the tension goes down and out, from top to bottom, face to feet, systematically, deliberately.

MIND TO BODY

Now we come to a facet of human relaxation that is inescapable: the relationship of mind to body, or the psychosomatic nature of humans. The mind and body are interacting, one helping or hindering the other. It is probably impossible to relax the body completely if the mind is under tension. Likewise, it is impossible to relax the mind completely if the body is under tension. This is observed also in animals in their need to concentrate during labor and the temporary viciousness of laboring animals if this concentration is disrupted in any way.

We have been stressing deliberate "do-nothingness" of the body during uterine contractions. Can you similarly relax the mind, make it go blank, and "think nothingness"? No! It can't be done. It's like trying not to think of an elephant. If you can't think of nothing during moments of concentrated physical relaxation, then you must think of something.

What should your wife think about, how should she occupy her mind while relaxing her body? Her mother-in-law problem? The fight with the neighbors? The bills yet unpaid? Hardly conducive to relaxation! No, she might select the earliest and most pleasant memory from her childhood or perhaps a time or place you have been together and deliberately dwell on this happy experience. She should relive it in all its pleasant aspects, utilizing every known sensory function in her recall—sights, sounds, fragrances, touch, taste—to make it more real. Early childhood states of trust and total dependence on others were accompanied then by automatic physical relaxation—test the muscular relaxation of sleeping children.

Recalling and reliving happy days in the mind's eye during uterine contractions helps her to dissociate from the pulling feeling in her back and lower abdomen. It is also a wonderful prelude to sleep for her and, incidentally, you. It is an automatic turning off of the mental worries, doubts, and frustrations that beset the day, to allow both the mind and body to relax as efficiently as they did in early childhood—you can sleep "like a baby," if you put your mind to it.

Now, such mental focusing of attention or mental control takes careful concentration on the part of your wife. This is more easily achieved in familiar surroundings with familiar sounds. The maternity ward of a hospital, even the better ones, tends to be distracting. Some have installed background music to help achieve relaxation. This is all right as far as it goes; it's a step in the right direction, but we have found by actual experience that there is a "background music" that beats all others and there is no substitute for it. It is the familiar, beloved voice of a husband, a lover, gently, softly, endearingly whispering in his sweetheart's ear that same line of love gobbledygook that was instrumental in starting the whole business of babies in the first place!

This is where you come in as a husband, and, by heaven, you're the only one who can play this role. Other instructors can teach physical relaxation, but it takes a lover to teach true mental relaxation.

Early in my tumultuous career of getting hospital administrators to allow husbands throughout labor I was capitalizing on one particular husband being with his wife because he was a doctor, an M.D., and therefore was allowed back in "no-man's-land." After the birth was completed I had the radiant mother tell the superintendent her reaction to natural childbirth.

I asked her in his presence if she had really wanted her husband with her. She unhesitatingly stated, "Oh, I couldn't have gotten along without him." I then asked if this was because of his being a doctor. She replied, "No, that had nothing to do with it. I needed him because he is my lover, not my doctor."

Play the lover role, then, during the glorious climax to your act of love—the birth of your baby.

Superficially you may think such details quite trite, but experience has taught us to bring food trays into the labor room for the husband as well as the wife, as we have seen uncontrolled panic take the place of calm cooperation when we sent the husband out, even for a moment, to get a bite to eat. I feed both mother and coach because it just makes sense that you need additional calories if you are doing this kind of hard work. I have been criticized often for this. But research done at Jubilee Maternity Hospital in Belfast (*Times* [London], December 17, 1992) confirms that women who were allowed to eat had less painful labors, had faster labors, were less likely to need Pitocin or cesareans, and had more vigorous babies at birth.

One reason women in labor have been forbidden to eat was fear of aspiration—that is, an anesthetized woman choking on vomit. However, Doris Haire, president of the American Foundation for Maternal and Child Health (www.aimsusa.org), researched this topic and reported to me: "There is not a single documented case of aspiration in an individual who was properly anesthetized according to today's standard of anesthetic administration." Again, science is catching up to Mother Nature. Family-centered hospitals will knowingly take this into consideration.

Your wife will peacefully relive her happy memory undisturbed by the forces of the uterine contraction (or a boiler factory) if she has that familiar, loved background music of your voice and your presence to reassure and encourage her. If she wants music, choose it together and download it to an iPod or MP3 player, so she hears what she likes. She feels secure in your presence—or she wouldn't have married you in the first place.

HUSBAND IS BEST AS LABOR COACH

The irreplaceability of a husband as a labor coach was illustrated by an incident. I arrived in the labor room to do the initial check on one of our patients in labor. She had come in during busy office hours and since she was still in early labor, I had seen a few more patients in our nearby office before stopping in to see her. Shortly after I entered the room a uterine contraction began.

I observed facial tension and rather poor abdominal breathing, and started fussing over these departures from what she had been taught. Her husband rose from his chair at her side and much to my delight laid a reassuring hand on my shoulder and said, "Don't worry, Doc, she does just fine when you're not here."

I couldn't help laughing with them at the interfering element of my presence. To such efficient teamwork I merely reminded her if she felt like pushing (second stage), to push on two things—the hospital signal button first and her bottom second, at least to let me know when the baby was coming so I could build up my ego by catching it. I went back to the office to see waiting patients, thinking how a few hours spent in evening classes teaching husbands to be labor coaches paid off so well in saving doctors' and nurses' time in the course of labor.

COACH SETS THE MOOD FOR LABOR

Coaches have the responsibility to set the mood for labor. We tell them when they arrive at the hospital that they should enthusiastically and with conviction tell everyone they come in contact with, "My wife's doing great!" and "I am so proud of her"—frequently, to as many people as possible. Keep saying it and after a while, when the coach needs reassurance he will hear the nurses out in the hall saying "Isn't she doing great!" If you enter the hospital and act like you do not know what to do then you are open to lots of interference.

In order to have your wife relax with the required procedures, make sure you know what they are during your tour. One of them may be electronic fetal monitoring (EFM). Some couples ask their doctor if they can have intermittent fetal monitoring as long as everything is going normally. The hospital may want an initial ten-minute strip of electronic fetal monitoring for *their* reassurance. After that it can be taken off and done again every few hours. During this time Mom might want to spend some time walking, sitting on the toilet (reassuring for some women since the fluids that leak during contractions run into the toilet), showering (this can feel good especially if she is having backache), or wherever she feels comfortable. After a while, when the contractions are getting stronger, she might want to lie down and get settled.

The nurse may want to come in and if you are not ready, simply look at her and tell her, "I just got her settled . . . just got her settled." Most of the time the nurse will smile and back out of the room knowing that you are doing a great job, getting this mother settled and relaxed.

We have discussed at some length the beneficial effect on the mother (and doctor!) of having a husband with his wife during first-stage labor. Now, what of the effect on the husband? I wish every reader could ask that question of a husband who has known the anxious, lonely vigil of pacing the waiting-room floor with a previous baby and then received training and coached his wife during labor with a subsequent birth. Seek such men out and ask them, if you have the opportunity. They'll talk your arm off about the benefits of being a participant. I routinely ask the husband after the birth is completed if he'd rather have been out in the waiting room during the labor. I get many explosive comments: "Not on your life," "I'd have gone crazy out there," and so on.

Now back to our comparison of how animals conduct themselves in labor and how you can teach your wife to do likewise.

NEED FIVE

(Need Five) is the need for relaxed breathing. If you recall, in first-stage labor we observed animals breathing the same way as they do when asleep—with their abdomens. Because labor is what the term implies, hard work, the depth and rapidity of breathing will vary with the length and strength of the uterine contraction.

DEEP-SLEEP BREATHING

Your wife should also breathe in the same fashion that she does when deeply asleep. However, her depth and rate of breathing will gradually increase as the labor progresses.

ABDOMINAL BREATHING

Sleep breathing is technically diaphragmatic breathing. Because the abdomen is visible and the diaphragm is not, we usually refer to it as abdominal breathing. In a state of relaxation her abdomen will rise and fall as her diaphragm goes down (inspiration) and up (expiration).

Her diaphragm may be compared to the piston in an air pump—as it descends it pulls air in, as it rises it pushes the air out. You cannot see the diaphragm working, as it is a hidden muscle, domelike in shape, separating the abdominal cavity from the chest cavity. As it descends, the abdomen must necessarily rise. As the diaphragm rises, the abdomen will fall back down. If a mother should inadvertently hold her abdomen rigid, then diaphragmatic action is impossible and she must then expand her rib cage to allow air to enter her chest. A rigidly held abdomen also interferes with the dome of the uterus going forward during contraction to allow its full force to act directly against the cervix.

Here's where husbands again prove their usefulness. When the uterine muscle contracts, it is directly under the abdominal muscle, and unless a mother exercises self-control she will tend to tighten her abdominal muscle along with the uterine muscle. To her, especially with her eyes closed, she can't see the difference, and because of the close proximity of the two muscles she can't feel the difference.

In other words, you can tell what she is doing and she can't. Guide her and coach her until you see and feel that she is breathing properly—during a contraction. Under your guidance, she will learn to "relax or bulge" her abdomen out actively, deliberately, with each inspiration, and then let go and rhythmically let her abdomen drop back down with expiration. The weight of your hand laid lightly on her abdomen serves as a guide. She will feel the rhythm of giving your hand a ride on the waves, up and down, or a sensation that her abdomen is an accordion and she is rhythmically opening and closing it to affect the coming and going of air. Should she get mixed up and hold her abdomen down, necessitating expanding her rib cage, gently correct this by verbal and touch guidance.

CONTOUR-CHAIR POSITION

This type of coaching is most easily achieved in the propped-up contour-chair position, as you are better able to observe the movements of the abdomen. It is usually automatically done in the side position as in sleep at home. However, if she has trouble catching onto the rhythm, utilize the "contour chair" until her confusion is cleared up. You can then lower the bed and have her curl up on her side again.

Abdominal or diaphragmatic breathing can be rehearsed at home during the course of pregnancy. A semi-propped-up position on the sofa or bed, using a pillow or rolled blanket underneath the knees, to simulate the hospital bed in a cranked-up position, will probably prove most convenient. The commercial contour or lounge chair could also be used. Both you and your wife will find this deliberate breathing rather simple to perform before the onset of labor.

The effect of the uterine contraction in labor may be at first confusing to your wife. She may get the bewildering feeling that the uterine muscle is her abdominal muscle. Of course this isn't so—she has the same set of abdominal breathing muscles, capable of being utilized for such, whether the uterine muscle is contracting or not. The two groups are separate and work independently of each other, but she needs your guidance and objective analysis to help her distinguish between the two.

NEED SIX

The last observation of instinctive conduct (**Need Six**) is the need for closed eyes during first-stage labor. Again, this is probably relevant to the simple need to exclude visual distractions to allow concentration. It is just as necessary with your wife as it is with the cat having kittens or the dog having pups. She must literally tune in to her body and pay total attention to what she is doing (relaxation and abdominal breathing). Her labor is all encompassing and requires her full span of mental and physical powers.

In early labor she will close her eyes only during the actual time her uterus is contracting. As the "mountain gets steeper," requiring more and more of her attention, she will tend to keep her eyes closed even between contractions in order not to allow any distractions. In this phase do not attempt to draw her into the idle conversation that she so readily and cheerfully entered into during the foothills phase. Pay attention to her needs.

PHYSICAL CONTACT

Some women do not want physical contact if it distracts their attention. Such advances on your part are motivated by noble thoughts and a desire to let her know of your intentions, but because they are distracting her from her work she may, like the other animal mothers, snap at you—verbally, of course. I had trouble in my early career by not properly preparing husbands for this possibility and had several get their feelings hurt. They were only trying to help but didn't realize they were actually hindering their wives. I had to reassure them that this did not reflect alteration of love for them—this is evident even in animals. They may warn disturbing masters by snapping during labor, but their affection is unaltered when the job is done.

Along with the sleep-imitation aspect and the closed eyes, I will comment on another facial characteristic that is probably the only true total muscle relaxation—the "duh" look, mouth dropping open. Your observation of your wife deeply asleep will reveal parted lips and mouth breathing. A moment's reflection by any person will bring to mind the phenomenon of a rather awful taste in one's mouth upon awakening in the morning. It represents simply the drying-out effect of breathing through one's mouth during deep relaxed sleep. This is the largest and therefore easiest route for air to pass—it takes effort to force air through the narrower nasal passages—and in deep sleep the body is economizing on effort.

EFFICIENT AIR EXCHANGE

All labor involves efficient air exchange, and good athletes breathe through their mouths. Labor also produces the morning taste in the mouth, which makes the iced orange juice given to all natural-childbirth mothers and fathers a very pleasant experience.

LAUGHTER

Laughter is the one great distinguishing characteristic in natural-birth rooms, and I recall one patient who had us all laughing at the moment of birth, including, I assure you, her husband. It was her sixth child in practically as many years and all by this method. She firmly maintained that the only reason she got pregnant so often was to get this glass of iced orange juice, because it was the best drink she had ever tasted.

When the late Dr. Grantly Dick-Read of England honored us with a visit many years ago, he commented with a twinkle in his eye that they would never allow this practice in his country—at birth they gave "hot tea with plenty of 'sugah'!"

The first stage of labor has been arbitrarily defined as the period of cervical dilatation.

In animals we observed that prior to this phase they may get up and move about, change position, turn around, etc. Women tend to walk, labor dance (sway their hips to and fro), or pelvic rock. This helps to open the inlet of the pelvis, speeds labor, reduces pain perception, and allows the baby to position itself for this journey. In late first stage or transition phase women tend to settle down and stay in one preferred position and discontinue any extra movements. They also concentrate deeply on what they are doing and are quite uncommunicative. They will very definitely snap crossly at anyone or anything that tends to disturb their concentration during this stage.

STEEPEST PART

This is the steepest part of the mountain and there is great need to pay constant attention to what one is doing. Side or contour-chair positions are generally positions of choice at this time. You will find your wife completely uncommunicative during this period. No more idle chatter between contractions. The interval between contractions has now diminished until your wife seems to think there is no interval at all—one contraction seems to follow closely upon the other. Don't try to engage in conversation.

Continue the slow, low-voiced, gentle, monotonous talking, now nearly whispering, in her ear. Continue the gentle pressure of your hand on her abdomen to guide her breathing or pressure on her back—but no extras now. What subjective feelings is your wife experiencing? She has a progressively increasing feeling of pressure in her lower abdomen, back, and bottom. Her birth canal is gradually filling up with descent of the presenting part (that part coming first) of the baby, usually the baby's head. Because of the proximity of the rectum behind the birth canal (it's truly a next-door neighbor), it now feels fuller and fuller.

One patient described the sensation as feeling "constipateder and constipateder" as time goes on. Even before the cervix has completely opened, the baby gets lower and lower. This sensation your wife should interpret as progress. She needs to have been reassured in advance that such progressive pressure feelings mean she's getting somewhere and that such pressure is beneficial to both baby and mother. Soon she'll be over the hump of the mountain to the more gentle plateau that just precedes completion, and that glorious achievement will soon be realized.

The crescendo action of the uterus gives your wife very little time to gather her wits or self-control between contractions. She may tend to get little panicky feelings because of this. Reassure her in a calm, firm voice if she tends to lose self-control. Get the train back on the tracks if she tends to break the rhythm of what she has been doing. I think the most encouraging comment you can make is, "We'll be seeing our baby soon." Take her mind off the power of the contractions and on to the joy of seeing the baby.

ONE CONTRACTION AT A TIME

Remember she only has to take one contraction at a time. She is never asked to do more than one at a time. If your reassurance is not effective, call your Bradley teacher. Ask your doctor or nurse for reassurance. Note that women are vulnerable to suggestion at this time and generally respond positively to suggestions like, "You can do it"; "The birth is near"; "The stronger the contraction, the sooner the baby"; "Welcome the power of this contraction. You are doing a great job." This feeling is generally the shortest part of labor, sometimes only a few minutes.

REASSURE HER

However, suggestions of drugs, Pitocin or Cytotec augmentation, or cesarean may be accepted also even if the mother only needs reassurance and a few more minutes to pull herself together and get back on track. Check your *Bradley Method Student Workbook* for more suggestions on active coaching at this time. Anyone who knows birth is familiar with the panicky feeling of the transition stage and should be able to assist you in reassuring your wife. The calm patient will proudly recognize that the efficient close contractions, the increasing pressure in her uterus means, "Now we're getting somewhere."

Your wife can tell by the tendency she will feel to push or bear down that the actual passage of the baby (second stage) is imminent now. She will tend to be confused whether she should push now with her contractions. Old-timers—experienced natural-childbirth mothers who have consciously given birth previously—know jolly well when it's pushing time, and as a doctor I have learned it is a waste of time to check them, they know.

However, if this is your wife's first child or first one by natural childbirth, you may want to evaluate the situation. Does she really have the urge to push or does it come and go away? What is her emotional signpost? What stage of modesty does she have? She might be checked by the attending doctor, nurse, or midwife to be sure the cervix is fully dilated. This is compared to being sure the door is fully open before you drive the car out of the garage. If your wife gets the definite urge to push, and the doctor or nurse is not there at the moment, summon them by the signal of the bell. It may be confusing to your wife as to whether it is truly pushing time or not.

If the examination shows the cervix is not completely dilated, there might be no point in pushing quite yet—it might be ineffectual. She might try leaning into the contraction gently or she may be encouraged to continue her relaxation with her chin off her chest and her deep, rhythmical breathing for just a while longer until the door is completely open.

I have heard scare stories about women pushing too soon and the cervix tearing or swelling from the pressure. I have not encountered this in a trained, undrugged mother in my practice. Encourage her to tune in to her body. True pushing time is not subtle and if this is not it, the urge will really be here shortly.

In women having their first baby, the transition phase usually lasts longer. For those who have had previous babies it may be only a momentary phase and pass so quickly as to be unnoticed. In either case it is the shortest phase of labor, and your wife should be made cognizant of this before she enters labor. Then she will recognize it as the acme of accomplishment that ushers in the most satisfactory and rewarding of all stages, the part where the mother gets to "do something"—push—with her uterine contraction. It is far simpler to do something than to do nothing! A video available from our Academy titled *Bradley on Birthing* is used as a labor review in many Bradley classes.

At a Bradley BIRTHS conference (a gathering of Bradley teachers from around the world), Dr. Bradley told the audience that in the beginning he had been against home births, but he had changed his mind about home births when he saw how some hospitals ignored the natural process and couples with midwives could be responsible.

6

SECOND-STAGE LABOR AND BIRTH

Squatting and Pushing

The steepest part of the mountain has been climbed. Now you and your wife have gone over the hump and are traversing the more gradual plateau that precedes the summit. You can see the goal ahead. You will very soon get that magnificent view (of your baby) that your efforts have been directed toward.

I pray for the day when all hospitals will have a natural-childbirth wing set aside so that all husbands can bring cameras on their trip and take a picture of this magnificent view. Because of the total absence of anesthetists and gas machines in natural-birth rooms our hospital allowed "daddy pictures" at birth when we introduced natural childbirth. These photos, even though amateurishly taken by husbands, enrich the baby book—vividly proving to the growing child forever after the joy and happiness his birth brought to his mother and father. How nice to see these pictures and hear stories about how you were wanted in the first place.

SEND US PICTURES

Grateful husbands have given us copies of these pictures to be used in introducing the concepts of natural childbirth to the bewildered, frightened, inexperienced parents-to-be. When his wife is that happy, that radiantly beautiful at the moment of birth, why should a husband not share the experience? Ask your doctor to show you some of these pictures and study them with your wife. They are like picture postcards taken of the view at the summit of a mountain by experienced climbers. But they are only pictures of others' experiences. How much more meaningful it will be for you and your wife to actually climb the mountain and see for yourself.

These are the thoughts you can transmit to your wife now that she has achieved the plateau that precedes the summit—the pushing stage, the second stage of labor, the stage just before you see and hear your baby. In order that you manage this stage properly, let's make sure that you understand it completely. Through knowledge and understanding we achieve proper performance. Let's go back to our instructors—the cat having kittens, the dog having pups—and carefully observe their actions so that we may then apply them to ours.

Up to now the animal has carefully imitated sleep—in location, position, appearance, breathing, etc. When the mother animal's cervix completely opens, allowing the baby to slip out of the uterus down into the birth canal (vagina), the baby pushes against a set of muscles called the levator ani group. This pressure sets up a reflex nearly identical to that set up by peristaltic movements of the colon pushing its contents down into the lower rectum, producing the urgency to have a bowel movement.

I do not know why the Creator unaesthetically put the cervix and vagina or baby door in this particular location—between the bladder and the rectum. It has necessitated a very unladylike but definitely mother-like position—squatting—to perform the act of giving birth.

UTERUS AND RECTUM COMPARISON

Whether we like it or not, the act of emptying the uterus is mechanically identical to emptying the rectum. As a man I will never know what it actually feels like having a baby. Being very interested in subjectively preparing mothers-to-be so they will know in advance what it feels like, I have asked this question, by questionnaire and verbally, of thousands of experienced natural-childbirth mothers, whose clear minds, unclouded by medication, know perfectly well what it feels like. I have always received the same answer: "It feels like having a big bowel movement."

We noticed in the animal mothers that when the cervix dilates completely and the baby descends against this set of muscles the animals change automatically from sleep imitation to "having a bowel movement" action. That is, they curve their backs, hold their breath, and make expulsive grunting noises. They follow the urge or signal given by the descent of the baby with appropriate action.

"GOTTA GO" URGE

This natural urge is also followed automatically by even untrained human mothers. We refer to it as the "gotta go" urge, or in some surprised, untrained mothers who acted involuntarily, the "Oh my gosh, I just did" action. I recall seeing a mother in consultation because her cervix hadn't completely dilated. It had opened to eight centimeters and remained there for quite a long time without progressing. Probably as a result of the calming influence of the specialist being introduced and the verbal exchange of reassuring pleasantries while I was donning a sterile glove to examine her, she became relaxed enough to allow the baby's head to slip through the cervix.

I never did do the examination. I didn't have to. The young mother got this startled look on her face, involuntarily held her breath for a moment, and, apologizing profusely, begged me not to pull the sheet down to examine her until the nurse had cleaned her up because she had "just done something right in bed that I haven't done since I was a baby!" She was gently reminded that the feeling was actually due to the descent of the baby. I assured her that she didn't need the examination now, that it was obvious her cervix had just finished dilating, and coached her how to squat, hold her breath, and more efficiently do what she had just inadvertently partially done—push her baby down. Her gratitude was heartwarming.

Animals in second-stage labor, then, act, look, and breathe as though they are having a bowel movement. So what should your wife do after her cervix is completely open and the baby begins to slip through? She should do the same thing. Now, here again, we run into the minor structural differences between humans and animals. They are minor but important.

You will have made a careful study of how your wife conducts herself in sleep for management of the first-stage labor. Must you now make a similar study in the bathroom and see how your wife manages a bowel movement? Definitely not. For two reasons: one is she just might resent such invasion of her privacy, and the other reason is she's not conducting herself correctly there anyway. This isn't her fault, it's the fault of so-called civilization and the invention of toilets. These gadgets designed erroneously to make it easier for human beings have probably been instrumental in keeping proctologists (rectal specialists) in business.

SQUATTING

This point was brought to my mind rather emphatically early in my specialty training by having made the acquaintance of a young doctor from India who had come to this country and to the same university for postgraduate specialty training. I found him a fascinating chap and we became close friends. One day we entered the men's restroom together and to my amazement he climbed up on the American toilet with his feet on the lid and assumed the squatting position. At my sarcastic jibes he countered with the statement that in his country people properly squatted to move their bowels and that in his medical training in India he had not observed hemorrhoids; he had to come to my country to find these abnormalities. We got into a heated discussion of what constituted civilization. I frankly didn't believe his statement that the bathroom facilities in his lavish home in India consisted of openings on the level floor over which one squatted.

I'm sure his mother in India was most bewildered when she received a request in his next letter that she photograph their bathroom and send the picture along, but she obligingly did so and thus helped to educate this backward foreigner.

I grudgingly came to the conclusion that he was right. The human body is so designed that the farther back the legs go the less flesh there is in the way of obstructing the downward passage of a bowel movement or a baby! A moment's serious thought would serve to illustrate this in contemplating children, prior to their introduction to toilets. I was giving a prenatal class a few years ago and covering this particular subject. We keep this introductory class as informal as possible.

While I was talking, one of the restless little toddler children in the group, diaper clad and not toilet trained, was ambling in front of me. Just at this appropriate moment the child stopped, squatted perfectly, held his breath, got red in the face as he, obvious to all, had a bowel movement in his diaper. There couldn't have been a better illustration of my topic and it gained a round of applause from the group.

No, labor coach, the bathroom fixture confuses the principles. Rather, let us visualize the proper position your wife should assume based upon observation of children, people of the Orient, or you yourself on a hunting trip out in the woods with no toilets around. This position is the squatting position and by now should be very familiar to both you and your wife as you have coached her to perform it many times in her household duties during pregnancy. (See Chapter 7.)

If the attending doctor, physician's assistant, nurse, or midwife has found by examination that the cervix is open—and if your wife is experienced on the subjective manifestations of labor and knows on her own that this is truly pushing time—then you should coach her to assume this full squatting position. From her standpoint it could more easily be done on the floor, as at home during her pregnancy. This may be inconvenient for the attendants but many now encourage this because it is so efficient. True squatting is the natural position for giving birth but can be assisted by squatting support devices on many hospital beds.

CONTOUR-CHAIR POSITION

In the latter portion of first stage and during transition stage many mothers find the contour-chair, propped-up position most comfortable. A few mothers may still be on their sides when the cervix opens completely. The mother's legs can be drawn back and apart, and she can roll her back up while on her side and give birth to her baby. This position is used successfully in home births and flat beds. Another position, for hospital labor beds, is the semi-squatting position. The bed can be positioned in a semi-sitting position, and we have found this quite convenient for squatting in second stage.

If your wife chooses the contour-chair position, we suggest you adjust the bed up and have her assume it. It provides a restful position between contractions in second stage. During contractions she should curl her back, pulling her head and shoulders forward (trying to peer over her pregnant tummy) by drawing her knees back and apart with her arm muscles. Her elbows should be thrust out and each wrist and forearm securely locked behind and under her knees. In this position during her downward pushing she should let her leg muscles be completely relaxed as she pulls with her arms. This allows her thighs to get adequately apart and farther back, serving to get the flesh between her legs (the inner upper part of her thighs) out of the way of the baby so it can descend. This action literally serves to shorten and open the birth canal or vagina.

HOSPITAL BIRTHING OPTIONS INCREASE

Today babies are born in the labor room; or LDR (labor delivery recovery) room; birth-room bed; or on the delivery-room table. It helps greatly if the beds are propped up like a contour chair, and if the delivery table is tilted with the head up and the foot downward. The degree of tilt should be nearly to the point of letting the mother slide down, almost a 45-degree angle. If your doctor is not oriented to natural-childbirth principles, make the request during pregnancy to have the delivery-room table tilted downward.

DRUGS LIMIT POSITIONS

When heavy anesthetics are used, the hospital custom is to tilt the table with the head down, bottom up. This is to attempt to make vomitus or secretions from the nose and mouth drain by gravity away from the air opening in mothers who are put to sleep. Natural-childbirth mothers find this upside-down position ridiculous and a hindrance to conscious expulsion of the baby. They say it's like trying to have a BM using a bedpan in a flat bed—trying to go uphill to do a downhill job.

DELIVERY-ROOM TABLE

When the delivery-room table is used (which is more often than most people think) it is usually an unadjustable flat affair. When this is necessary, utilize two pillows—one under the mother's shoulders, one under her head for support. As she pushes with contractions, you as a coach can help immeasurably by pushing the pillows so that they follow her curled back forward. The best adjustable back support remains an educated, pillow-adjusting husband.

A modification of the husband's support of his wife is to use the two pillows to rest on between pushes and have the husband hold his wife with his arm directly around her shoulder or a bit lower across the wife's back, depending on where she likes support, his cheek against hers as he lifts her forward and supports her not only physically but also emotionally by hugging her. One of our patients requested this, as she wanted to feel her husband, not our "darn pillows." Her request was happily granted.

When an LDR room is not available and this is your wife's first baby, there will be time enough in second stage to perform for a while in the labor-room bed. If this is not her first baby, she will probably be moved to the delivery (birth) room shortly after reaching second stage, or some doctors may even want her moved there before she starts pushing, if she has had several previous babies. If a birth room or LDR room is available, then no move is necessary.

We have covered the position of second-stage labor in the imitation of bowel movement action. Whereas we had six points of performance to follow in first-stage labor, we have only three in the simple action of second stage. The first is position, squatting; the second is breath holding; the third is pushing or bearing down.

SECOND-STAGE PERFORMANCE NEEDS

POSITION

Knees back, elbows up and out, chin on chest.

The second-stage squatting position involves all these things. Other positions can be adapted but you need to keep these three things in mind.

1. Knees back, if the mother is on the floor in the squatting position this happens automatically. Other positions require attention. The mother should put her forearms, not just her hands, under her legs and pull the legs back toward her ears. It is not necessary to have the knees far apart. This assures us that the mother's back is rounded like a ball and the baby

comes sliding out—like on a slide. When the mother is holding her legs they should be loose and relaxed. Next, we have the mother take a deep breath, which fills her lungs and creates a cushion of air that pushes the uterus forward and downward. This cushion encourages the uterus to come forward getting the baby into the proper alignment with the pelvis.

2. Next, the mother puts her chin on her chest, which traps the air and increases the inter-abdominal pressure. You can try this yourself (Mom or Dad) right now. Take a deep breath of air and look up at the ceiling and push down with your abdominal muscles and let the air out and relax. Now take a deep breath of air and roll your shoulders over, putting your chin on your chest and push down with your abdominal muscles—then let your air out and relax. Think about it, you probably found that putting your chin on your chest created greater abdominal pressure. This pressure helps the baby to be born.

3. Elbows up and out. This seems like it has nothing to do with birthing, but in effect the position with elbows up and out can make a big difference in whether the mother's perineum tears or not. When the elbows are down (at your sides, pulling your legs apart) there is a great deal of extra pressure on the mother's perineum and she is more likely to tear. If an episiotomy is performed, it is more likely to extend because of the extra pressure caused by having her elbows down— which pulls her legs out, instead of back. When the mother has her elbows up and out, away from her body—the knees come back, and there is generally enough room for the baby to come out, most of the time without tearing or cutting. Having the knees back causes the baby's head to create pressure that numbs the perineum. If a pressure episiotomy is needed, and the numbing has occurred, it can be done and the mother does not feel it. Many mothers have told us that the burning sensation that sometimes occurs at birth is stopped or reduced when they get their knees back, elbows up and out.

Put all of these points together about second-stage position and the natural position would be squatting. That is the ideal, but sometimes compromise is acceptable. An imitation of the squatting position is called the classic position and is vastly better than the old lithotomy (flat on the back with the legs up in stirrups) position. The old position led to many serious tears and much pain and suffering after the birth.

BREATH CONTROL

You will note that anyone moving his bowels does so by holding his breath during the act. Your wife, then, should be an efficient breath holder during her uterine contractions in second-stage labor. Her breath control now is totally different from first stage. For the two stages of labor the conduct is very different indeed. In order for her to hold her breath during as much of each contraction as she feels comfortable holding—she is going to need all the breath her lungs can hold. Therefore, instead of the gentle abdominal breaths of the first stage, she should be encouraged now to breathe large, deep breaths.

"ATHLETIC BREATHING"
I think a good comparison for our term "athletic breathing" in second stage is an underwater swimming race. The swimmer plans to exert his energies for as long as possible on one breath, underwater, to see who can swim the farthest. Whoever wins the race will be dependent upon how thoroughly he fills his lungs with air before he is called upon to hold it.

In quiet breathing there is a lot of unused stale reserve air present. This stale air must be "washed out" by deeply inhaling and exhaling first. The efficient swimmer would fill up completely, empty out completely several times to rid the lungs of stale air, and completely replace with fresh. In labor, this also helps a woman wait to push until the contraction is strong.

BEGINNING OF CONTRACTION
When your wife feels her uterine contraction beginning she should calmly inhale as fully as possible three times. The first

two lungfuls should be completely emptied out by totally exhaling. The third big breath is the one she should hold, at the height of inspiration, with her lungs fully filled with fresh air. She should calmly hold this full breath and simultaneously hump over, chin on chest, put her forearms behind and under her knees, and, elbows out sideways, pull with strong arm action until her limp, relaxed legs come back as far as they can. Some women have second-stage contractions that begin so suddenly they only have time to take one full breath and start pushing.

When she has held this breath as long as she comfortably can (there is no need to act heroic and try to hold beyond comfort or count), she should exhale completely. If, at this time, the uterine contraction is still present, she should immediately inhale completely and hold this second time as long as the breath holds out. She should then exhale again completely, emptying all of the air, and in the rare instance that the uterus is still working, she could repeat another big inhalation and hold this—until the contraction lets up. If she is surprised by a contraction that is very strong from the beginning, she takes a deep breath, gets into position, and holds from the very beginning. All breathing is open-mouthed with an open, relaxed throat.

REST PERIODS

During the rest periods between contractions she should let her legs slip back on the elevated foot of the bed, or if she is on a flat delivery-room table, into the metal supports provided for holding the legs during rest periods. One of the fundamentals for the consciously cooperating mother is that she should never be restricted in any way. Her arms and legs should not be bound down by straps or held in any position against her will as are those of uncooperative medicated patients. This is a must that should be clearly understood and agreed upon in advance by the doctor and his attendants.

NATURAL URGES

Bradley mothers push and hold their breath according to their natural urges. They do not pant, or pant-pant-blow, candle blow, or hee hee breathe, etc., because these artificial breathing patterns can lead quickly to hyperventilation (a loss of carbon dioxide [CO_2]). Hyperventilation changes the acid-alkaline balance (pH) in the body instantaneously, causing mother and baby to go into distress. CO_2 is a waste product produced in the body, normally, and is also the gas that tells humans when to breathe. A low level of CO_2 tricks the body into believing it doesn't need to breathe. The baby needs to be born from a mother in normal respiratory status.

PUSHING

The third point of performance for your wife in the second stage of labor is the muscular action of pushing. Again, unaesthetic as it may be, this muscular action is identical in performance to that of being constipated and squatting out in the woods with the firm determination of moving one's bowels. Breaking down the details of action, it involves downward action of the abdominal muscles while holding the diaphragm (breathing muscle) immobile via breath holding, so that the increase in intra-abdominal pressure is directed downward and out the flexible opening of the vagina. Simultaneously, this muscle-surrounded aperture, the vagina, should be deliberately opened by consciously relaxing the circular, or sphincter, muscles that surround it. These circular muscles, when tightened, tend to draw the vagina upward and closed. When relaxed, the vagina descends downward and open.

KEGEL MUSCLE

For unknown reasons, which again only the Creator can clear up, this set of muscles is also part of and controlled by the same muscles that open or close the bladder (in front) and the rectum (in back). Anatomically this is a single muscle divided into three component parts in women. It is called the pubococcygeus muscle, as it passes from the pubic bone (in front) to the coccygeal bone (behind). However, it has circular parts that surround the urethra (bladder opening) in front, vagina in the middle, and anal sphincter (rectal opening) in the back.

For simplicity and out of respect for the late Dr. Arnold Kegel, who first described its importance, we refer to this muscle as the Kegel muscle and put great emphasis on its utilization.

While your wife is pushing down she should deliberately relax this muscle at the same time that she is tightening her abdominal and arm muscles. The purpose is, of course, to aid in opening the vagina for the passage of the baby. You, as a coach, can help her by reminding her as she pushes to try to urinate, try to move her bowels, and relax her Kegel muscle.

The perineum should be flat or bulging forward. This means the mother has relaxed her Kegel muscle. If it is being pulled inward, the mother is doing a Kegel contraction and playing tug-of-war between the Kegel and the uterus. The uterus is stronger and will win but it may take longer and be more painful. Especially during contractions let the Kegel go, let it relax and birth becomes easier.

A woman who holds back by tightening this muscle for fear she might release urine or fecal matter is also holding back her baby, and instead of pushing the baby down and out is merely playing tug-of-war with her own sets of muscles and is ineffectually squeezing the baby and causing herself a lot of unnecessary pain.

We have tried discontinuing the routine enema given as part of the prep on admission in labor. I doubt very much whether it is necessary, actually, from a physical standpoint. However, from a psychological standpoint it may be helpful in some cases. We find some mothers push down more effectively if they know their rectum is empty. They seem to have a psychological hesitancy to move their bowels in this exposed position, probably a carryover from childhood toilet training.

REDUCED BLADDER PROBLEMS

Another of the many benefits of natural childbirth is the small number of bladder problems afterward. There is no need for catheters before, during, or after the birth of a baby, only from the delivery of a baby. No matter how careful and sterile the technique of catheterization, it is an undignified, miserable feeling, traumatizing to some degree the urinary passageway as well as introducing existing bacteria from the outside to the inside of the bladder.

GO HOME TWO HOURS AFTER GIVING BIRTH

A new obstetrical patient of mine who had had both previous babies with anesthetics was told that with natural childbirth she could go home with her baby anytime she wished, after two hours from birth (if she breast-fed). She asked if we did house calls to catheterize our patients! Such a possibility had never occurred to us—it had never been needed. Mothers who can empty their vaginas themselves can certainly empty their bladders themselves.

We encourage the husband to encourage his wife to deliberately wet the bed while pushing. We joke to the couples that, after all, the laundry is paid for here and patients don't have to rinse out a thing during their visit. The "open door policy" must prevail during pushing, and in order to get one door to open all three must be opened.

In second-stage labor, before the baby is actually coming outside the mother's body, that is, during its descent down through the internal portions of the birth canal, your wife's face will have about the same appearance as that of a piano mover who is intermittently called upon to lift a heavy piano, hold it for a minute, then set it down, rest and chat for a few minutes, then lift it up and hold it some more. Her face will get a reddish color during this breath holding (as did the little toddler's at the prenatal class), and her features will be contorted in the same way that piano mover's are—with effort, not pain. Please, please do not confuse these two.

I recall a "stubborn Dutchman," as his wife referred to him, who was very skeptical over his active role. He actually wanted no part of being a participant in the birth. Out of due respect to our many wonderful Dutch-descended patients, he had reasons. Darn good reasons. When I noticed his reluctance to attend classes preparing him as a coach, I inquired why.

His frank answer was revealing. "Doc, I sat out in that waiting room for hours with the other two. I could hear her screaming through two sets of closed doors, and they told me they were giving her all the medicine they dared. Doc, I get sick to my stomach when I hear her scream and realize I got her pregnant."

After receiving a "guarantee" that he could leave anytime he saw or heard anything that upset him, he reluctantly took the course. As he told us later, he simply didn't believe a word of natural childbirth, he came only because his wife pushed him into it.

His wife was an intelligent, earnest woman who I just knew would be a good obstetrical athlete, and she was. During first-stage labor he sat fidgeting on the edge of his chair and looked so much like a little boy waiting for his first piano recital that his wife giggled. With gentle coaching she performed beautifully in the labor room, and, under the circumstances, so did he.

When the cervix was nearly dilated I suggested now that he accompany his wife to the delivery room for the actual birth. He panicked completely. He could still hear those screams from the other times. His wife said, "Oh, come on, this is different," but he still held out. As the nurse took the calm mother to the delivery room, I took the panic-stricken husband through the two sets of doors to the waiting room. On the way I had him help me prop the doors open, both sets. Then as he sat shakily in the waiting room I asked him when his wife began screaming to feel free to get up and close the doors. However, in case he didn't hear any screams, he was still cordially invited to join his wife if he wished. Fortunately there were no other births going on that night. His wife was magnificent. We chatted between pushes. She kept giggling over her husband's fears.

He heard the chatter and giggles from his distant waiting room, but no screams. Finally loneliness and curiosity got the best of him and he came carefully around the corner, unfortunately just at the moment she was pushing hard with a contraction. As he saw her contorted red face (effort!) he panicked the second time, ran up to her, and begged, "Take the gas, honey! Take the gas!"

She stopped pushing long enough to say, "Oh, get away, I'm busy!" Then in a few seconds she finished her push, looked up at his distraught face, and saved the whole situation by laughing uproariously at how he looked. This chagrined, but finally convinced, honest Dutchman became one of those so-called (by opponents) fanatics for the benefits of natural childbirth. I'm sure he would resent being called fanatical, because he could see and hear the difference between a medicated maniac and the same beloved woman as a calm, trained athlete who could interrupt her work just to kid him. It is significant how often these so-called fanatics for natural childbirth are people who have experienced medicated, untrained childbirth first. Why aren't they fanatics for medicated deliveries?

EFFORT, NOT PAIN, ON HER FACE

Don't confuse the facial appearance of effort with that of pain. The more pressure your wife applies to her bottom, the better she feels and the better the baby will cry and expand its lungs at birth. This rhythmical intermittent mother pressure was meant to be, for both mother and baby.

TESTING THE PRINCIPLES

Again, let me throw in the challenge of testing the principles of the method. After you have satisfactorily coached your wife to take three big breaths, hold the third, squat, and try to move her bowels, ask her not to do any one of the three—see if there is a difference! Don't just *believe* natural childbirth, try it.

PRESSURE LESSENS PAIN SENSATION

Pressure on human flesh makes that area devoid of pain sensation—in proportion to the amount applied. You will find your wife earnestly pushing hard—for the simple reason that the harder she pushes, the better she feels. Why? Because pain perception is dependent upon circulating blood to the involved area, and pressure slows down or stops the circulation momentarily. This is really nothing new. The next time you see someone whack his shin accidentally on some object, watch what he does. He doesn't just look at his shin and say, "Oh, fudge," but will grab the shin and hold it in a tight grasp until it feels better.

The oldest anesthetic known to the battle surgeon was a tourniquet. Many a leg has been amputated painlessly without any anesthetic other than a properly applied tourniquet to stop circulation to the area involved. This occurs not only on the battlefield. There was a news article about a forgetful but clever (I thought) intern who made an emergency run in an ambulance but forgot to take along his instruments (this is not apparently limited to plumbers). A man had had his leg mashed in an elevator accident and needed an immediate amputation. The intern borrowed a policeman's belt and club and applied an improvised tourniquet. With only this anesthetic he amputated the limb (probably with a borrowed knife!), for which the victim calmly thanked him.

Many a time I have called up to the patient to stop cheating by letting air out her nose. One husband asked in bewilderment how I knew what her nose was doing when I was watching the other end. I couldn't see her nose from my view. The answer is really quite simple: While she was properly pushing, the area around her vagina blanched white from the pressure. When she let air out her nose the pressure was momentarily lessened and the circulation returned to this area, which turned red. This didn't feel good and she would hold her breath again. I told her husband her bottom looked like a signal light blinking white and red, which informed me what she was doing. She laughed and pushed steadily instead of intermittently from then on.

Mothers who have had previous children do not have to push as hard, or as long, with subsequent births. We do not want a "champagne cork" effect, the baby popping out, so mothers are instructed to push only hard enough to effect descent. Experienced natural-childbirth mothers can assess the rate of descent and calmly "ooze" the baby out slowly and gently.

YOUR BODY AUTOMATICALLY LETS YOU KNOW TO BREATHE

A few critics of natural childbirth claim breath holding is harmful to the baby, depriving it of oxygen. There is no clinical evidence that imitating animals can harm a baby. If the mother's oxygen gets low, she automatically replenishes it with another breath so that neither mother nor baby is depleted. As an observer you will notice that the time interval between contractions, which shortened to practically nothing in the crescendo or transition phase, now, in second stage, lengthens out again. The rest period becomes longer between contractions, when the mother is called upon to work actively with her uterus.

This is a very nice arrangement, as it gives the mother time to catch her breath and her self-control, enabling her to push more effectively. It also brings back a return of her communicability. Whereas in transition phase she became nonverbal as she concentrated on her work, in second stage she may resume her talking between contractions; there's time enough now. Recalling the mountain-climbing comparison, you two are now traversing the more gradual plateau that leads to the summit, and there is time for pleasantries. She may ask you to perform little tasks such as wiping her brow with a cold cloth, moistening her lips, and adjusting the pillows more to her satisfaction.

CROWNING

As the baby begins to "crown," that is, stretch the external vaginal lips until they surround its head like a crown, your wife may exhibit a change in her reactions to what's going on. She now knows by the way it feels (the external skin is more sensitive to feeling) that the baby is actually coming out and that the long-awaited moment is here. Women act differently at this moment. Some women describe this as a burning sensation. Others say it is an exciting, provocative feeling. I think it is best described, and the emotions that accompany it, as a "birth climax" that compares the high emotional content favorably with the sensations a woman feels in reaching a full sexual orgasm with the man she loves.

Your wife may, as she feels the baby coming out, give a little squeal of ecstasy. She may cry out in surprise over the momentary new sensation of the baby passing through the external lips. This is probably related to the fact that the clitoris, which is at the front of the vagina, where the minor lips come together and surround it, is now being stimulated by the passage of the baby, giving a definite sensual feeling to this moment. It is only a momentary fleeting feeling. Some women make no outcry at all (as is true in sexual orgasms). It is attended with great emotional feeling either way. I have observed mothers spontaneously wrapping their arms around their husband's neck, kissing, crying with joy, squealing with delight, and so on. I always feel like an intruder and outsider to an intimate relationship between husband and wife. I would feel embarrassed if the husband weren't there!

One mother gave us a very complete description of the sensations of birth. The bowel-movement comparison was during the gradual descent of the baby as it traversed the internal vaginal canal. The rectum is located between the descending baby's head and the forward curving lower portion of the backbone (sacrum). The pressure from the downward-sliding baby is manifested against the rectum, due to the unyielding nature of the backbone behind it and the physical phenomenon of going around a curve. We refer to the lovely curve of the derriere of ladies as the "baby sliding board." It is very similar to those playground sliding boards in schoolyards as it curves forward and upward in the lower half, and both were made for children to traverse.

In descending, the baby, after it has gone around the curve of the sacrum, comes forward as it actually leaves the mother's body and places tension and pressure—for the first time and only momentarily, at the actual moment of passage—in the clitoral region. In a sexual climax this is the area that receives and gives vigorous pressure as part of the ecstasy experience. At the moment our patient's baby was born, her husband told her afterward that she made sounds just as she did during orgasm.

Could this experience between two people who love each other combined with the thrilling privilege of seeing for the first time the product of their blended love—their baby—be related to the nuisance they make ever after to be together when subsequent babies are to be born? Experienced natural-childbirth parents are never nonchalant in their desire to share this event. Husbands have been known to leave no stones unturned in their determination to be with their wives—e.g., the college student who chained himself to his wife in labor, the legally oriented ones who have applied injunctions and legal restraints over their physical exclusion from delivery rooms, and others of like nature.

One of our highly intelligent husbands, Terence Cory, a news writer for ABC-TV and the father of two children, had been an excellent labor coach, very happy and satisfied with the good show his wife, Ginny, put on under his direction. He was not a fanatic for natural childbirth—that is, not until he moved to Chicago and his wife became pregnant again. He found out, to his fury, that the state of Illinois still had backward, old laws (purposeful in the "knock 'em out, drag 'em out" era) that ignored and defeated all principles of family-centered childbirth. He became a fanatic in a very short time. A man of action and connected with the TV industry, he decided his contribution would be to have a public debate on TV between professional people advocating natural childbirth with husbands as active participants, and those professional people who were against these concepts.

I warned him that those against would decline an open debate, as the public is on the other side, and it's an uncomfortable position to assume. However, he was determined to try. Try he did, but the show went on with only those advocating the principles present; the others declined. Their negative part was voiced by the interviewer and cut to ribbons by the enthusiastic advocates.

Today Chicago is one of the best places to give birth naturally. Dr. William White—son of the late Dr. Gregory J. White, the author of *Emergency Childbirth*—and Dr. Mayer Eisenstein each have active home birth practices in Chicago. Dr. Eisenstein has written a book called *The Home Birth Advantage*. Their enthusiasm and passion for natural family birthing is contagious.

In 1947 I first experimented with these concepts and ran up against opposition from nearly all angles—other doctors, hospital administrators, nursing supervisors, and others. I made a prediction then that troublesome as the necessary changes in obstetrical management inherent in natural childbirth may be, we were dealing not with minor techniques of management but with major human rights, human rights that seem superficially simple and obvious—the right of a woman to bear her children with all her mental faculties and her husband present, if she wishes. Whether the medical profession liked these concepts or not, they would have them jammed down their reluctant throats by public demand. This was met with laughter then. The laughter has faded now.

We have had patients fly to Denver from California in order to have babies with their husbands participating. However, the following quote from the *AMA News* of January 1, 1965, indicates that young husbands and fathers-to-be once faced possible consequences before they invaded delivery rooms.

DELIVERY ROOM "INVADER" FINED

A New Jersey father who gained unauthorized admission to a hospital's delivery room in an attempt to witness the birth of his second child was told by a Union, N.J., County Court judge that the incident will cost the father a substantial fine.

Judge Ervin S. Fulop upheld a conviction and fine by Plainfield Municipal Court Magistrate Warren J. Lynch against John O. Keim, 33, on charges that he acted in a disorderly manner when he refused to leave his wife's side in the delivery room at Plainfield's Muhlenberg Hospital. In appealing, Keim contended that he had caused no trouble and that he did not know three men, summoned to the delivery room to ask him to leave, were policemen.

A hospital nurse had told the Municipal Court that she notified Keim that layman fathers were not permitted into the delivery room under hospital regulations, but only into the labor room. Mrs. Iris Keim was moved quickly to the delivery room after her arrival at the hospital. The nurse said that Keim's insistence on going into the delivery room led her to give him surgical garb while permission was asked for him to be admitted.

When the request was denied and Keim entered anyway, just moments after his daughter had been born, the nurse phoned the police. Three policemen wearing surgical clothing went in the delivery room, but Keim reportedly still would not leave. He told the court that an earlier pregnancy of his wife ended in a miscarriage, that his wife had German measles during the recent pregnancy, and that she was two weeks late in delivering this child.

Most hospitals today not only allow but encourage the father to be present.

FINAL PUSH

Now, back to the birth room and your role as a coach. After the final push, accompanied by surprised squeals of delight, get your heads together. Put your head down with your wife's, cheek to cheek. Hold her hand—she's through pushing with it—love her, praise her, share her joy. Actually, I don't need to direct you to do this. If you're there, you just can't help but share her joy; it is contagious to all present but particularly to the one who loves her. I have seen tears of shared joy unashamedly in the eyes of husbands at this moment.

SKIN TO SKIN

After the baby is born, put the baby (skin to skin) to the breast and hold, touch, and rub the baby. If the umbilical cord is too short for the baby to reach the breast, which is unusual, the mother and father may caress the baby while it lies crosswise on the mother's lower abdomen. We feel this is a substitute for the animal mother's licking her baby. This serves as a dermal reflex. It is amazing how many babies void or empty their bladders upon this stimulation. It has been reported in animals that if babies are deprived of this stimulation at birth, the kidneys do not function.

CONSIDERED A BLESSING

Down through the ages, to be wet upon by a newborn was considered a blessing. We are delighted to know the kidneys work and indeed consider it a blessing. It is during this time the parents discover what the sex of the baby is, assuming that they did not know ahead of time. Sometimes people who *think* they know get surprised. Medical testing is sometimes inaccurate. More and more midwives and doctors just hand the baby to the parents without telling them this. Making the discovery yourselves is a great joy!

BABY TO THE BREAST IMMEDIATELY . . .
SKIN TO SKIN

After the mother puts the baby to her breast, mother skin touching baby skin, the attending nurse puts a warm baby blanket over the baby and the mother. The baby should be skin to skin with the mother. During labor and birth the mother was working very hard and she is very hot. The human body produces radiant heat that warms the baby as long as it is skin to skin with Mom. Wrapping the baby in a blanket shields the baby from its mom's heat, actually causing it to cool down and get cold. The result may be placing the baby in a warmer, separated from its mother. The mother should put her hands directly on the baby, gently massaging it under the covers, never through them!

FLUID IN THE LUNGS

Should the baby be extra "juicy," or have extra fluid in the lungs, the doctor or midwife may hold it upside down for a moment to help drain the fluid. Your doctor or midwife may use a bulb syringe to suck the mucus and salt water out of your baby's nose and mouth—they may also be tilting the baby's head backward to let gravity assist in draining the nose, sinuses, and mouth. In unmedicated births, however, this is seldom necessary. During the natural process as the baby descends into the birth canal its head passes the pubococcygeous muscle and then the perineum. The perineum stays close to the baby's head, face, shoulders, chest. When the baby's chest passes the perineum, the perineum pushes against the baby's diaphragm and causes what is called the "fetal Heimlich maneuver" as uniquely captured in our Bradley video *Giving Birth . . . Naturally*. This pressure causes the baby to spit out the fluid and mucus in its mouth and throat making suctioning rarely necessary.

CHANGES IN THE BABY

Internally, miracles are happening to your baby. Valves are automatically closing in the umbilicus to prevent baby blood from running back in the cord. Valves are closing in the baby's heart, valves that remained open during the intrauterine life to direct blood through the cord and placenta to pick up oxygen and nourishment from the mother via the placental surface. Other valves that remained closed are now opening for the first time, allowing the blood that used to go to the placenta for oxygen to circulate through the baby's lungs, which now contain air for the first time. Isn't it a miracle that these parts know how to do these things at the proper time?

BABY'S FIRST TIME APPEARANCE

If you have never seen a newborn baby before, I think it would be beneficial to know in advance what to expect. The skin is a pinky-purple hue at birth. The blue element comes from the normal fact that the baby has extra blood at birth. This is a leftover from the intrauterine life where the extra blood was necessary, as it got its oxygen secondhand from its mother's blood. This extra blood will gradually be disposed of, which gives the baby a normal yellowish or jaundiced color about its third day of life. At the moment of birth it imparts a bluish tint, which, when combined with the red color of a healthy baby, gives a pinky-purple result.

PUFFINESS

Also, when babies are just born there is a layer of built-in fat just under the skin together with a normal state of puffiness of the skin (edema), which gives the baby's face a jowly, ponderous look. One mother told her husband all her newborn babies looked just the way he did in the mornings after a big party.

SQUINT

The baby has been in darkness for nine months, and the sudden introduction to light makes him squint. Another mother said newborn babies looked to her like Mr. Magoo, the nearsighted cartoon character. After a period of adjustment the baby will open his eyes. Do not expect some preconceived color of your baby's eyes at birth—they are all gray-blue and achieve adult colors later.

BABY'S HEAD

The baby's head may appear elongated and perhaps just a little lopsided. Don't worry about it; it's supposed to look like that due to the molding effect of its position in the birth canal. There may be a little puffy area of the scalp, usually to one side of the dome, which is called the "cap of birth" and comes from the gradual dilatation of the cervix. All these little irregularities will gradually fade out in a few days and are normal.

SKIN

Newborn babies' skin will be wet with salt water and have irregular blotches of grayish-yellow material here and there, which we dub "baby cold cream." It is actually accumulated skin oil and has the impressive name vernix caseosa. Long ago it was thought to have magical properties and was carefully saved and used for multiple purposes, medical and otherwise. One use was for gun collectors to rub on gun stocks as a special wood preservative. Vernix can simply be rubbed into the baby, it is beneficial and protective. Your baby does not need to be washed or scrubbed clean, it already is clean.

HAIR COLOR

Do not jump to conclusions about the color or consistency of the baby's hair. It is wet with salt water and may appear curly when it actually isn't. We refer to newborn babies' hair as "puppy fuzz" because it is so fine and, as with puppies, the color at birth may change somewhat later.

EPISIOTOMY

If the doctor has done an episiotomy while your wife was pushing—and no anesthetic other than pressure and whiteness of the flesh being cut is necessary—he will inject Novocain in the edges of the cut and put in the necessary few stitches while you and your wife are counting fingers and toes and playing with the baby. The coach may then be asked to cut the umbilical cord after waiting for at least half an hour or more following a natural birth.

BREAST-FEEDING OR SIMPLY BONDING

The baby may or may not be particularly interested in eating immediately. He will like the warmth of your wife's breast and nurse when he is ready to receive a sticky substance called colostrum, which precedes breast milk. The American Academy of Pediatrics has called colostrum "nature's vaccine for the newborn"—that is, it provides nourishment, immunities to protect your baby, and a laxative to get the digestive system going. (The sooner the meconium, or first stool, is passed, the fewer problems we have with jaundice.) A major beneficiary of the first breast-feeding will be your wife. The uterus contracts by reflex from breast stimulation, which also helps to separate the placenta from its contact with the uterus. The contractions further help to reduce the size of the uterus to nonpregnant proportions, and serve to shut off the maternal blood vessels that formerly fed the baby.

THIRD STAGE OF LABOR

Your wife will feel the placenta slip out of the uterus and down into her vagina from five to ten minutes or more after the birth.

Breast stimulation by the baby causes hormone production, which assists the placenta in coming out. Sometimes the mother is asked to bear down and expel it.

The passage of the placenta is called the third stage of labor. Animals instinctively eat their placentas after they are passed. Some animal mothers chew the cord in two, at a safe distance from the baby. We watch for the cord lengthening, which indicates the placenta has separated and is ready to come out. If it hasn't, we wait a while, if the mother is doing well, patience is important. Pulling or tugging on the cord too soon can be dangerous. When it has separated from the uterus, your wife will have a full feeling in her vagina, followed by a delightfully empty feeling, as the doctor lifts the placenta out by traction on the cord. Her big tummy is now fully emptied of the baby, the water, and the "baby house," or placenta. We usually hear admiring comments from both husband and wife as they compare the size of the abdomen now with the size it was a few minutes before.

If you want to see the placenta after your birth, ask for it to be washed off and shown to you.

The placenta is a magical organ that contains many undiscovered secrets of function and of secretions. The reason animals eat theirs is probably related to some substance it contains that serves to stimulate uterine contractions. Breast-feeding is the natural way to get the uterus to contract, but if your uterus is not contracting, your doctor may give you an injection of an oxytocic drug, which serves the same purpose. In early days, human placentas were said to have been dried, ground up, and compressed into pill form and fed to mothers postpartum.

Today, however, we have many good chemicals that serve the same purpose if needed. With our many enthusiastic breast-feeding mothers we generally do not need to give oxytocin; it depends on how well the uterus contracts. This varies with every mother and every pregnancy. We remind the parents (in the rare instance) when we give an oxytocin drug, usually Pitocin, it saves the mother the trouble of eating the placenta.

After the baby and placenta emerge and episiotomy stitches,

if any, are completed, the mother needs to drink iced orange juice to restore her depleted blood sugar that was used up by the uterine muscle action during the course of labor. It is, as we have mentioned, replacement of fluids used in labor, replacement of potassium, and also refreshing to the mouth, which has become quite dry from mouth breathing. In the spirit of sharing childbirth, we also offer the father a glass of iced orange juice with his wife as a little token of doctor gratitude. We refer to this as the refreshment served at the original birthday party.

Shortly after the baby is born and placenta expelled, your wife may experience a mild shaky, chilly sensation. This is not due to coldness or to nervousness as some mothers immediately assume. Rather it is due to the physiological changes in circulation. It is only a momentary phenomenon and is normal.

At this happy moment in two people's lives (or should it be three?), I teasingly state in a dry, matter-of-fact voice, "Next time I'll keep the husband away, put the mother to sleep, and deliver the baby myself." The opponents of natural childbirth should hear the assortment of return comments that invokes! Its prime purpose is to trigger grateful, sincere statements from the wife to the husband: "Honey, I don't know what I'd have done without you."

WALKING BACK FROM THE BIRTH ROOM

Walking back from the birth room has become associated with natural childbirth since its earliest inception. It is not necessary, and if the mother has labored during usual sleep hours we do not advise it. (Of course, if she has had medication or complications, it is out of the question.) However, we have had thousands of mothers who insist on walking back and quite frankly take delight in doing so. The other day, in the wee small hours of morning, one of our repeat mothers gave birth, and because of the hour I suggested she ride back to her room. She saucily stuck her tongue out at me and walked out of the room with her beaming husband.

I find it hard to argue with these obstetrical athletes. It's equally hard to *find* them as I make hospital rounds—they simply don't stay in bed; they keep insisting they are not sick, so why should they stay in bed?

In hospitals that do not yet have birthing rooms, any doctor who utilizes affiliated Bradley Method childbirth educators to prepare his or her patients in natural childbirth, I give fair warning, will be resented by his or her colleagues as a patient stealer. Many hospitals have recovery rooms on obstetrical floors where all patients are taken for a two-hour period after they have babies. The exuberant natural-childbirth mothers look so good, feel so good, and act so happy that the medicated or anesthetic-recovering ones ask them, "How come?" In that two-hour stay with several other patients in the same room, believe me, they find out how come. Having once experienced natural childbirth, the parents, I have noticed, are never reluctant to talk about it.

ENTHUSIASTIC PARENTS

The greatest handicap we have found in practicing natural childbirth has always been the overenthusiasm of our patients. Of course, it's a two-edged sword, and if medicated patients looked, felt, and acted better than nonmedicated ones, the promotion would be for the other side.

7

THE COACH'S TRAINING RULES

Coaches do not function only during the game. They are essential in the physical preparation of the body during training long before the game. They also prepare the athlete's mind so that there is a clear conception and understanding of the duties involved. By their interest and enthusiasm they should be a living symbol to the spirit of the player, motivating the individual to want to play the game at her level best.

The same applies to the role of husband and coach, to help your wife prepare like an obstetrical athlete for the great event—labor and the birth of this child.

Why bother? Why let all this new rigmarole possibly interfere with your golf game? Women have babies; that's their job!

TRAINING AN OBSTETRICAL ATHLETE

Coaches, imagine that someone offers you one billion dollars, tax free, if you can convince your wife to complete a marathon run. What would you do? First of all you would have to make sure she knows this would benefit her also. Perhaps promise her some of the money, tell her she would be in fantastic shape and able to accomplish something that would make her proud. If she is overwhelmed remind her that the rules are that you only need to complete the run. Placing is not an issue. Now what? Training and preparation are the keys.

WELL NOURISHED . . . EVERY DAY

You would want to make sure she is well nourished every day. She needs extra sleep because she is training for a marathon. Keep stress out of her life so she can pay attention to this event. Ensure physical training so she has the stamina necessary and the right muscles prepared and ready to go. Build her confidence so she knows and believes she can do this. Help take care of her day and night. Massaging those sore muscles. Walking with her. Talking to her. Letting her know you care about her. Would it be worth it? A billion dollars is a lot of money. A baby is worth more, much more, than a billion dollars. This may be one of the most important, memorable events in your life. Help her out.

IN PAIRS FOR A REASON

Parents come in pairs. If you think the only task you have as a parent is to get your wife pregnant, you're going to be like the farmer who thinks all there is to farming is planting seeds. You will harvest only the weeds of resentment to your passivity. You are poorly prepared for parenthood and have yet to recognize your responsibilities. Your schooling didn't prepare you—they teach typing, tap dancing, and tomfoolery, but precious little preparation for parenthood. Your parents probably didn't prepare you. No one ever prepared them—they cannot pass on to you what they didn't receive. The rising divorce rate, the rejection of parenthood, and the increase of child abuse reflect what pitiful examples of parenthood many couples are.

Maybe I'm old-fashioned, but don't kid yourself, the hand

that rocks the cradle still rules the world, and always will. Motherly women and fatherly men acting as wholesome symbols of strength and righteousness in a family setting of mutual love and respect continue to be essential to progress in any civilization.

PREGNANCY AND BIRTH STRENGTHEN BONDS

The reaction your wife has to her pregnancy and the birth of your child will reflect on the relationship between you as husband and wife, and it will reflect on the relationship between mother and child forever after. Will she look upon childbearing as a horrifying ordeal that ruined her figure and seared her soul? Will she recover from an anesthetic with a curse on her lips— "Never again; you have the next one"?

Or will she joyfully share with you even the little nuisances involved and thank you for getting her pregnant, and bless her God for the privilege of being a woman and of giving birth? I recall one trained young mother who squealed in delight at the moment of birth, "That was fun!" Then she added, as she ecstatically kissed her husband, "Oh, honey, when can we have another one?"

I hadn't had time to dry off this baby and she was looking forward already to the next. These are the mothers with actively participating husbands whose understanding and encouragement of their wives constitute the most important factors in natural childbirth.

YOUR PARTNERSHIP IS FOR LIFE . . .
BE THERE FOR EVERY EVENT

You are going to live with this woman until "death do us part." How rich, full, and meaningful that life will be is very much dependent upon your ability as a participant in parenthood. This does not exclude but takes precedence over the golf game, pool hall, poker game, CD player, computer, etc. Let's get on with it. What are your responsibilities as a coach?

PHYSICAL CONDITIONING

I'm sure you have had similar experiences, but let me use one of mine to illustrate a point. I had been away from the old hometown for eight years attending school. On a nostalgic return to visit relatives and old friends, I happened to meet the woman who had been judged the prettiest girl in our high school class. I had to be told who she was, and even then found it hard to believe. I remembered her as a beautiful, poised girl, whose sparkling eyes reflected the joy of living. I now saw before me a swaybacked, round-shouldered, sagging, varicose-veined woman whose dull, listless face reflected the boredom of life. I exclaimed in amazement to a friend, "What happened to her?" His answer: "Oh, she's had several babies since you last saw her and they just ruined her."

BABIES DON'T RUIN MOTHERS

I take vigorous exception to this statement. No baby ever ruined any woman; mothers ruin themselves! Don't keep blaming the innocent babies.

Now, unfortunately, you can't in all honesty blame the woman entirely. One must blame society and ignorance. Having babies need not ruin a mother's life.

BEAUTIFUL NATURAL-CHILDBIRTH MOTHERS

There are thousands of beautiful natural-childbirth mothers whose lives remain beautiful after many babies. Many childbirth educators, having had many babies apiece, attest to this fact. They serve not only as teachers but also as shining examples. On an invited lecture tour in Ottawa, Canada, I had the pleasure of sitting with Dick Hartman, the young husband of one natural-childbirth mother (a Canadian R.N.). We both beamed with pride watching his leotard-clad wife, Rhondda, on a TV program, as she showed how housework and baby care could be done in a beneficial "mother-like" way.

Her confidence, slim body, and good posture spoke more than

words, and she had had two babies and was in early pregnancy with her third! She now has had five babies without drugs and is just as beautiful. Her book on exercises is a classic in the field of natural childbirth: *Exercises for True Natural Childbirth*. There are some things your wife can do and some ways of doing those things that will preserve physical and spiritual beauty. These things do not necessarily fit Emily Post's way of being "ladylike" but rather the natural-childbirth concept of being "mother-like."

PRENATAL EXERCISES

The term "exercises" tends to immediately tire some women by its very connotation. I would prefer to call them "body mechanisms of pregnancy." Most of them are simply ways of doing daily tasks. Our fervent plea is, try them! Your wife really needs your help and encouragement. Being motherly is not the norm. She may need to be reminded, encouraged, and reassured to act mother-like in the privacy of her home.

It is not the intention of this book to teach your wife how to do these important exercises, rather to teach you as a husband why they are important and how you can help.

THREE WAYS

Your wife can learn them in three ways—by going to Bradley natural-childbirth classes, where they are demonstrated and performed, by studying a text, or by doing both. The first is, of course, far preferable, but if no classes are available in your locality, don't give up. Contact the headquarters of The Bradley Method (www. bradleybirth.com, 1-800-4-A-BIRTH or 1-818-788-6662) to find a local Bradley teacher who can provide classes and support.

BRADLEY CLASSES ARE VERY IMPORTANT

The motivation in wanting you and your wife to actually participate in childbirth classes is twofold. First, I think the exercises are easier for her to learn if she observes the teacher doing them and then has the teacher observe her doing them. The second motivation is that although these classes provide "physical training" for natural childbirth, they actually cover all aspects of natural childbirth, including what you need to know to be a great coach. One cannot completely divorce the body from the mind. There is a great psychological benefit from association with other experienced natural-childbirth couples.

Let's assume your wife knows how to do these exercises from either classes or books. Now, as a man, you will want to know enough about them so that you can help your wife know if she is doing them properly, and, most important, understand the logic and reasoning behind them.

AN ATHLETIC EVENT

Let's not lose sight of the coming event—labor and birth—as an athletic event. It is this in a very true sense. Let's repeat again, it's darned hard work, and the term "labor" is most appropriate. The amount of energy involved is comparable to what a football player uses playing a full game of football, offense and defense.

A player who entered such a game without having had any recent experience or taken any special training to condition the muscles involved would be so stiff and sore and miserable after the game was over that he probably would have to be carried from the field.

NINE MONTHS OF PREP TIME . . .
NOT JUST TWELVE WEEKS FOR CLASSES

Similarly, a mother, given nine months' notice of game time, who makes no physical preparation, yet when the whistle blows must play the full game (there is no substitution here), would have to be carried from the field and would do well if she could walk comfortably within several days thereafter.

Conversely, an athlete who takes cognizance of the physical conditioning of the muscles involved and performs daily training exercises during these preliminary months to get in condition has no trouble walking off the field when the game is over. A physically prepared natural-childbirth mother often makes a nuisance of herself (to hospital attendants, that is) by walking back from the birth room.

BACK, BELLY, AND BOTTOM

The muscles involved in your obstetrical athlete are the three B's—Back, Belly, and Bottom. These are the ones that must be strengthened and made flexible, and have the stiffness of disuse worked out of them by daily calisthenics—just as for any other athlete.

BASIC PREGNANCY EXERCISES

Let's begin with the ones that do not represent any expenditure of extra time on her part, but rather are simply mother-like ways of doing what she's going to be doing anyway.

TAILOR SITTING

This could hardly be called an exercise, as it represents an inactivity, yet it can be done in such a way that it will stretch and make flexible the muscles on her bottom and the inner aspects of her thighs that will allow her to put her legs farther apart in second-stage labor—or open wider when the time comes.

This approved and appropriate way for her to sit used to be thought of as unladylike, but today we know how important it is. Join her on the floor, read or watch TV with her.

It is called "tailor sitting," or "Indian style," or "kid sitting." It should preferably be done on a hard surface like the floor so the crossed feet will be on the same level as the hips. Your wife should lean forward and put her elbows on her knees and enjoy talking, music, writing, watching TV, etc. This serves to let her enlarging uterus fall freely forward (where it belongs!) instead of tipping backward (where it doesn't belong). The leaning forward bends the bow (her back) and thereby loosens the bowstring (her abdominal muscles), thus allowing the uterus room to come forward. Some mothers find that putting a pillow under the back part of their hips helps them to feel comfortable sitting this way.

The principles behind this position of sitting can be illustrated in many ways. First, it's the most comfortable way there is to sit. Let any child alone and he will not sit in a chair with his legs together, and if you turn your back he won't stay there long, you'll find. It's uncomfortable. Kids are far more comfortable sitting on the floor—reading the funny papers or books. If left alone, they will continue to do this automatically even up to teen age.

Tailors have sat that way since time immemorial for the simple reason they sit all the time in their work and found this position the most comfortable way there is to sit.

It is a natural way to sit, as manifested in Native Americans, Africans, Chinese, Japanese—it is seen in the entire Orient and much of the rest of the world.

CHAIRS LEAD TO MORE PROBLEMS

Among these peoples, varicose veins of the legs, hemorrhoids, uterine prolapses (fallen wombs), etc., occur far less often than they do in Westernized countries where people are forced by custom to sit in chairs. This is not the only factor involved, of course, but it is an important one.

Sitting erect in a chair or, even worse, slumped back in a chair will make your wife's uterus descend deeply into the pelvis instead of freely falling forward. These positions contribute to posterior labor (back labor). It compresses the large blood vessels going to the kidneys and legs and interferes with circulation to these parts.

LEG PROXIMITY

Then, adding insult to injury, someone long ago decreed that ladies do not sit with their legs apart—that it is ladylike to cross the legs! Ah, brother, we do have problems.

I am not asking your wife to assume a sprawl in public but, rather, am giving voice to the first great commandment for pregnant women: thou shalt not sit in a chair in private. You can help by understanding the importance of this exercise. Pregnant couples should sit on the floor to eat meals off the coffee table as often as possible. If any tasks such as studying, reading, talking on the phone, crafts, or perhaps peeling potatoes are normally performed standing up or sitting in a chair, these can be done sitting on the floor tailor-fashion. Remember, however, that no one should sit in any position, including our approved one, for great lengths of time. Long periods of inactivity make for poor circulation and stiff muscles.

In the later months of pregnancy, when her uterus is quite large, it is permissible, for short periods of time, for her to sit contour-chair style with her legs sprawled comfortably apart and elevated higher than her hips. Ordinary lawn chairs of the contour variety serve well for this purpose, or using pillows or blankets to lend appropriate support on the sofa is nice. The uterus is so large it tends to fall forward from its own weight, even in this sensitizing position. Variety in position also serves to make a break in the monotony. It should be obvious that your wife should wear flexible or loose-fitting garments that allow complete freedom of movement.

SQUATTING

Your wife will have many occasions to get down to do something. If you have no children as yet, this would be in getting a pan out of the lower shelf in the kitchen, picking up around the house, gardening, and so on. I once checked on a housewife without children to see how many occasions she had to "get down" in the course of one day—it was about twenty-five. I then observed a young mother with small children and it was over a hundred times!

Squatting may be awkward at work, but is possible in the ladies' lounge, or with slacks on to pick up a sheet of paper or get supplies from a low file cabinet.

This is your wife's magnificent opportunity to prepare the muscles in all three B's—Back, Belly, and Bottom—on a daily basis. Squatting is, again, unladylike, especially the way the teacher will show your wife to rise from this position—tail first!

Squatting increases the outlet diameter of the pelvis and reduces the chance of needing a cesarean section.

Again, you don't have to attend a special class to have this simple, natural way of doing something (getting down and back up) demonstrated. Just watch a small child at play. The little girl toddler will comfortably squat for long periods (it's a natural position) while playing with her dolls, or jacks, or what have you. (So did your wife when she was that age and her squatting muscles didn't protest one bit.) When the little toddler rises she comes up from the squat tail first and then straightens all the way up. So did your wife at that age, and pregnancy commandment number two is: so shall she now! Coach's training rules.

REMIND HER TO SQUAT

If your wife is bending over to pick things up and keeping her legs locked straight and bending her back—jamming her pregnant uterus deeper in the pelvis, misusing her lower back muscles that alone must support the pelvic contents—remind her to squat.

IMPORTANCE OF SQUATTING

There are many reasons why squatting is important in pregnancy. The first is that the squatting position is the most effective pushing position in second stage. If her muscles are so stiff from disuse and unfamiliarity with this position that she cannot properly assume it, the baby may need more time and pressure to come down the birth canal. It is the physical means of opening the door to let the baby out.

The second reason is the importance of the physical factor of legs apart and back to let a baby out. It's not good for the baby to be held back.

We always instruct our patients that if they are ever caught inadvertently with a baby knocking at the baby door, wanting to get out, to push the baby out. It matters not who is around or where they may be at the time. Police, letter carriers, firefighters, taxi drivers, grandmothers, and Boy Scouts (both with and without a first-aid badge) have been known to "deliver" babies under emergency nonhospital situations, and two results stand out significantly as a consequence: (1) how well the mother gets along, and (2) how well the baby gets along.

DELIVER
Isn't that a silly word, "deliver"? Would it deflate the ego of the attendant at such a birth if it were pointed out that both mother and baby would have done fine if left alone?

Would it hurt their pride if it were pointed out that umbilical cords don't have to be cut and tied at all, that it's better just to leave them alone and intact?

YEARS OF NON-USE TAKES TIME TO STRENGTHEN
Back to the legs-apart business. What if a woman, through cultural tradition or ignorance, has never, since early childhood, sat with her legs apart? What if these muscles are so stiff from disuse that she can only put her legs halfway apart? If she can only open the door halfway it's going to take longer and hurt more than if she were capable of opening the door all the way. What if unfounded anxieties, resulting from negative conditioning for years, make her afraid to spread her legs apart and back to let the baby out? She's afraid it will hurt to let the baby pass. No one ever convinced her in advance that the exact opposite is true: it hurts the mother and the baby if legs are not spread apart and back!

The squatting position is important. Help your wife as she becomes acquainted with it and gets more so as her pregnancy progresses.

No, your wife doesn't have to squat on the ground or floor at the moment of birth—although there is no good mechanical reason why she couldn't have a baby there, except it's a bit unhandy for the doctor, midwife, and nurse, and floors aren't noted for being the cleanest of receptacles for newborn babies.

SQUATTING ON DIFFERENT SURFACES
We can still use the birthing bed or delivery table, but we also still use the squatting position on it. This is accomplished by

having the mother squat on the bed or using the classic position by tilting the table forward (they're adjustable) as far as is convenient and propping up your wife's curved back with pillows, or with that favorite of adjustable back supports, a knowledgeable, cooperating husband. Some beds have squatting bars and some women insist on squatting on the bed or floor with a clean blanket under them.

SOME BATHROOMS STILL NEED YOU TO SQUAT TO USE

Friends traveling worldwide have told me stories of bathrooms that consist of a hole in the floor that you squat over. At one of our informal prenatal meetings a husband interrupted to describe a scene he had observed in China during World War II. He was riding as a passenger in a military convoy. He noted a woman worker interrupt her work momentarily, squat by the side of the field, give birth to a baby, place it in a sling on her back, and return to work—completing the entire affair while the convoy was passing!

Your wife will not want to go around squatting just to be squatting. It is merely a sensible way of getting down and back up when she has occasion in her daily life to do this, for instance, working in the flower garden, talking to you, or picking up something light. If the two of you are snapping green beans together, take them from the sink and put them on the floor to snap them. Instead of that misery-producing half bend over the sink she'll be keeping her back straight and bending her legs, squatting on the floor, to perform the same task. The Creator put hinges at the knees and hips, not on the back; your wife should use these hinges. Straight backs and bent legs never harmed any pregnant woman. Straight legs and bent backs have harmed many.

PULLING OR ACHING FEELING

Some pregnant women will complain of a pulling or aching feeling in the inner thighs when first performing their squatting exercise, especially so if it has been years and years since their bodies have assumed this position. This is not a sign that all is lost and they can't do what others do.

TENNIS . . . ACHY MUSCLES AT FIRST

If one hasn't played tennis for years, then plays a vigorous game, the tennis-playing muscles may ache at first. This is not a sign to give up tennis but rather a sign that one should play more frequently for shorter periods of time. This calls to mind the boy who combed his hair only once a year—it was so painful he couldn't understand how anyone could stand to do it once each day. Older mothers may be less flexible. Or it may not be age at all, but rather the type of activity the mother usually does. The executive who has worked in an office for years with her legs crossed, sitting in a chair, will find that she is stiff and some muscles complain when she first starts her squatting exercises, regardless of her age. This does not mean she can't be a mother; it means her daily activity now, in pregnancy, must include the mother-like squat position at short intervals. These intervals can gradually be lengthened each day as the muscles regain their lost flexibility.

FERTILITY CLOCK

I recall one lady, years ago, who decided frantically at near-menopause in her late forties that she had missed something by never having had a baby. This was brought to her with a jolt when her menses became irregular—the first sign to her that her days of fertility were numbered. Her life had been so busy with her career that she hadn't paid much attention to having a baby; that is, until the warning sign appeared that soon she couldn't. That did it, she wanted one, right away! Her first question was, "Do you think I'm too old to have one?" Although warned that older women have a slightly higher percentage of abnormal babies, she was determined to take her chances. I assured her that, with a bit of assistance, her body could be conditioned adequately to give birth. It would take a bit of doing, for she was overweight, had borderline high blood pressure, varicose veins, and poor circulation in her legs from years of office work. Nevertheless, it could be done.

PHYSICALLY, NOT PSYCHOLOGICALLY, SPIRITUALLY, OR ECONOMICALLY

The ideal physical age for a healthy young woman to give birth is about fourteen years of age. This is not the ideal age psychologically, spiritually, or economically, but it is physically. Pregnant girls this age do not really need additional instructions in exercises. Why? They've been doing them anyway without instructions—tailor sitting, squatting, pelvic rocking, regular vigorous physical expenditure of energy in many ways. Even just talking on the phone in the privacy of the home teenagers go through practically the whole gamut of our approved body positions before the conversation is over, as their parents can inform you. I have had obstetrical cases from eleven years of age on up; their problems are many, but none are related to muscular rigidity.

Well, we laid down the law to our middle-aged career woman with no ifs or maybes. She was sincere and so was her husband. It took about everything in our infertility bag of tricks, and they were blessed with success. Her husband was given an extra dose of coach instruction and the impression that we meant business. She was never to sit in a chair. She was never to cross her legs. She was never to bend her back when she could bend her legs. She was placed on a well-balanced high-protein diet, and she stuck to it. Results? During the course of her pregnancy her body fat gradually reduced, her blood pressure came down to normal, the circulation was better established in her legs, and she performed in labor as efficiently as a teenager. Her posture was improved and she actually sparkled with joy. Her husband sobbed with happiness at the sight and sound of their baby at birth. He kept saying, "I thought I would never see one of my own." There wasn't a dry eye in the room from empathy with these people's happiness. She never had another menstrual period afterward—it was to be their only. That was years ago. Their daughter is a lovely dark-haired woman with large dark eyes who used to come by the office regularly to say hello before I retired.

The personal rewards of obstetrics are multiple. Obstetricians jokingly maintain to other specialists that ours is the only creative aspect of medicine; the rest is just repair work! You don't have to be a teenager to do natural childbirth, but the older you are, the more you need its benefits.

PELVIC ROCKING

Your wife will be instructed in horizontal pelvic rocking, which is lifting (not arching) and relaxing her lower back rhythmically while on hands and knees. At first you think she has lost her mind, acting like a four-legged animal down on all fours wagging her tail—up and down, though, not back and forth.

Let's start from scratch and reconsider a few facts. We are studying lower animals to see if we can glean from them how it is possible for them to give birth spontaneously without medication. The anatomical differences between people and, say, cats, dogs, horses, and cows are relatively trivial. The anatomical similarities are so remarkable that as premedical students we can study their bodies to gain knowledge about our own.

ON THE FARM

Having been reared in a farming environment with familiarity of these species, I cannot recall ever seeing varicose veins, swollen ankles, hemorrhoids, fallen wombs, or convulsing mothers among animals. These things I first met in the study of human beings. If their bodies are so similar in structure to ours, why don't they have these things? Why do not the milk cow's hind legs swell and get broken-down veins as she bears calves repeatedly each fertility cycle? I wonder what your wife's body would eventually look like if she also bore a child repeatedly every cycle from the onset to the cessation of her fertility.

What's the main physical difference between these animals and your wife? Somebody taught your wife at a very early age to walk on her hind legs, that's what. Her internal organs are all still suspended in little ligamentary hammocks from her backbone, just like the four-legged animals. These internal organs include her uterus—which is suspended from her lower back (sacrum) by the uterosacral ligaments.

ORGANS THEN CAN FALL FREELY

When the backbone is parallel to the ground these organs fall freely forward. When the backbone is perpendicular to the ground, the organs fall downward and inward where, frankly, they weren't designed to be. The heavy, enlarging uterus compresses the blood vessels and interferes with circulation to the legs and kidneys. It stretches its own supporting ligaments out of shape and weakens the back at their point of attachment. A woman has been defined as a "biped with a backache," and she has reasons! The nonpregnant uterus weighs about one-half to three-quarters of a pound. In the short course of nine months it and its contents increase in size until it weighs fifteen to twenty pounds. This means the ligaments attached to the lower back are going to be calling on the spinal muscles of this area to do twenty times more work in these short nine months.

STRENGTHEN NOT BIND

Now, if the leg muscles were to be called upon to run twenty times farther or faster at the end of a nine-month period, how would an athlete prepare them? By binding them with rubber bands? By trying to do their work for them? Would that tend to strengthen them steadily? Of course this is ridiculous. Doing their work for them would tend only to weaken them progressively, as it would any muscle anywhere.

Then what in the world is the logic behind girdles and binders designed to do the work of the uterine-supporting muscles? Aren't they equally ridiculous and don't they serve to progressively weaken muscles that should be progressively strengthened?

In our office, "girdle" is a swearword. Recognizing the abysmal insanity of fads and customs, we only scream in protest the first time a woman wears one (even if it is in the form of abdominal support in panty hose). From that point on we either swear, weep, or both if we find it again.

Now, if your wife has a physical deformity of her back or abdomen and an orthopedic specialist has prescribed an orthopedic artificial supporting device for good sound medical reasons, that is another matter. What we are dealing with here is healthy women.

Let's get back to that athlete who needs to strengthen his leg muscles to do twenty times more work. How will he do it? Not by rubber bands but by exercise—daily, regular exercise. Each day he will exercise a little longer, each time to the point of full fatigue. Each day the muscles would get stronger and stronger. Each day the point of fatigue will get further and further along. The blacksmith develops such strong bicep muscles by using them daily, not by compressing them daily with rubber bands. The same advice goes for your wife's back and belly muscles— she should use them, not squeeze them!

DOUBLE PURPOSE

The pelvic rocking exercise, on all fours, serves a double purpose. It makes a temporary four-legged animal out of a two-legged one, and it actively exercises the lower-back and abdominal muscles, which need to be strengthened to support the increasing weight of the offspring growing in her uterus.

MAKE IT A ROUTINE

If this is your wife's first pregnancy, she should perform this exercise just prior to retiring each night—until the beginning of the seventh month. From that time on she should do as women who have had previous children do from the very first knowledge they're pregnant: perform it at midmorning (ten a.m.), after lunch (at noon), and midafternoon (three p.m.) as well as before retiring. Many women will be able to do this at work if they have an office with a door they can shut. Others might not be able to perform during working hours. They should do pelvic rocking as soon as they get home.

After each episode of pelvic rocking they are to lie down in the "running position" on their side, top leg drawn up, back curled comfortably forward, to let the heavy uterus remain forward for a rest period of ten minutes at least, or longer if they are tired or not pressed for time. How long should your wife do this pelvic "tail-wag"? During the busy daytime episodes we usually specify forty wags.

DOUBLE AT BEDTIME

At bedtime this number should be doubled with a rest period between the wagging episodes—her hips reclining against her heels, hands and arms folded before her as a pillow for her head. This is called the "froggy" position of rest. It is actually quite comfortable and is the position babies frequently assume in their crib—bottoms up, head to one side, knees drawn all the way up, hands above or under head. One of our teenage mothers found it so comfortable that she dozed off and awakened the next morning still in the same position. Most older women will feel muscle-stretching sensations in their thighs and hips in this position and should stay this way just long enough to catch their breath, then get back up on all fours and pelvic rock again, forty more rocks, then crawl into bed.

TO THE POINT OF TIREDNESS

In my early years of practice I did not specify the number of pelvic rocks, insisting that the patients should do it to the point of tiredness, then quit. I altered this suggestion when I got a phone call at midnight from one of our teenage patients. She said, "Doc, I've been doing pelvic rocks since nine o'clock but I'm not tired. Shall I keep it up?" Youth is a wonderful thing, isn't it? Our older patients or those with sedentary jobs may find fatigue at first before they reach the prescribed number. Of course it's all right to stop and rest when tired. The back muscles will gradually strengthen with time, regardless of age, until the less limber are as capable as the rest.

COUNTERACT ERECT POSTURE

The purpose of longer bedtime pelvic rocking is to counteract the erect posture during the day and to bring the uterus forward and upward from where it has descended. The other purpose of deliberately tiring these muscles at bedtime is obviously that she gets to rest afterward. Pelvic rocking need not be done on arising, as sleeping in the running position with the upper leg drawn up serves a similar purpose of allowing the heavy uterus to fall freely upward and forward. This is manifested by the decrease in swelling of the ankles and veins of the legs during the night.

Wayne Wright, the husband of one of our enthusiastic young patients, Carol Wright, an acrobatic dancer, proved his wife had paid close attention at the prenatal class where we stressed complications following the descent of the uterus. He brought in a picture he took of his wife on her due date, dressed in ballet leotard, walking around the kitchen at home—on her hands! Her graceful young body was quite capable of this even at full-term pregnancy.

If I were tired of being a teacher of natural childbirth, I would limit my practice of obstetrics to professional dancers. You should see them perform in labor! Magnificent breath control, relaxation, etc.—old stuff to them. This new mother pouted because I wouldn't let her walk back from the delivery room on her hands! She could have, and would have. The only reason I didn't allow it was the inevitable resentment from medical colleagues against our enthusiastic, exhibitionistic natural-childbirth patients. They create enough attention just walking back on their feet!

AS COACH . . . HELP HER BEFORE BED
Our suggestion: Before you get in bed each night, no matter how late it is or how tired you both may feel, help her with her pelvic rocking! How can you help? Try counting her wags for her while you rest on her side of the bed. That way, while she's rocking, you're making her side of the bed comfy and cozy for her. You could pelvic rock with her; it might be good for your back, too.

PELVIC ROCK SUMMARY
In summary, this hands-and-knees exercise looks strange but is temporarily making a four-legged animal out of your two-legged wife who has been parading around on her hind legs all day, al-

though her internal organs are designed and supported like
those of four-legged animals! Evolution hasn't caught up here as
yet. In order to prevent the development of varicose veins,
chronic back strain, fallen womb, toxemia of pregnancy from
decreased kidney circulation, etc., all of which are peculiar to
the erect posture, encourage your wife to perform this exercise
as directed.

SLEEP POSITION

Again, this could hardly be called an exercise, but it is so important we include it for emphasis. One of our new patients com-
plained of inability to sleep because her husband insisted she
sleep on her back so she wouldn't squash the baby. She was miserable with a backache.

BABY CAN HURT MOM . . . NOT MOM HURT BABY

Let me strongly reemphasize that a mother cannot hurt a baby
in the uterus by lying on it. It's the other way around. The baby
can hurt the mother by lying on her, especially as it gets larger.
Babies are suspended in salt water, which serves as an equalizer
of pressure. Any local pressure applied to a bag of water is immediately distributed equally and therefore harmlessly diminished—I believe it is a principle in hydraulics.

WATER BALLOON EXAMPLE

To illustrate this, one can fill a large, tough balloon full of water,
insert an inflated small, fragile balloon inside it, then try to
break the small one by striking the large one. Now, of course, if
you strike hard enough, you can injure the large one. Or putting
it another way, you can hurt a mother, but it is indeed hard to
hurt a baby. Even most nonpregnant women sleep on their abdomens or curled up in a ball on their sides.

During the early months of pregnancy they should continue
the same way. Those who sleep directly on their abdomen will
find, as pregnancy progresses, they are trying to balance themselves on a lopsided mountain. The side position with the top
leg drawn up and, especially in later pregnancy, supported on

something, is the preferable position. This "something" to support your wife's raised leg can readily be your own legs or perhaps an extra pillow.

Sleeping on your side with your back against your wife's abdomen is not only convenient for her but also allows you to feel the movements of your baby during the night. I find husbands intrigued by this movement if it is a first baby. The intrigue seems to fade with increasing numbers of children, probably related to increased need for rest. Having children is indeed hard work, but nothing compared with taking care of them. I have often joked with my patients that I've "had" about twenty-three thousand babies but, thank goodness, didn't have to take care of them.

From the waist up we are not so concerned what position your wife assumes in sleep. The side-relaxation position works well for most moms. Comfort is a primary concern. Warning: if the mother puts the pillow along the top of the bed and then puts their head on that pillow and her bottom arm behind her, then gets into the side relaxation position, she may find it uncomfortable. Solution: there is an easy fix. Just pull the pillow so it is at a 45-degree angle, so the mom can put her head on the pillow and have the pillow squished along her breast. Much more comfortable. From the waist down we are very concerned that she draw her top leg up and shift her hips over.

Some wives prefer to sprawl with their arms, others prefer to cuddle them under their head or shoulders—it doesn't particularly matter. The purpose of the drawn-up leg is to form a bony supporting "tent" between the leg bone, hip bone, and bed. This allows the uterus that has been "tail-wagged" out of the pelvis to fall freely away and forward and remain there during the sleeping hours.

You can realize how uncomfortable your wife would be in the later months of pregnancy flat on her back by imagining yourself trying to sleep in that position with a bowling ball lying on your abdomen. I think you would tend to turn on your side so that the bowling ball would fall away from you.

RETAINED WATER

Pregnant animals seldom show retained water in their body tissues, whereas pregnant humans do. This can come from naturally increased blood volume, in a healthy mother, or interference with kidney function. One way of interfering with disposal of water via the kidneys is for a pregnant woman to sleep on her back with her baby on top of her. It doesn't even have to be a baby. Tests were done on urine volume output in women whose uteri were enlarged due to fibroid tumors and not pregnancy.

OUTPUT DIMINISHED LYING ON BACK

The volume of urinary output was measured in the two different positions and found to be diminished whenever the woman lay on her back. Again, I know of no pregnant animal that spends the night balanced on her backbone with all four legs pointing skyward. This may be a factor in the absence of toxemia of pregnancy in lower animals.

Your sprawled-out pregnant wife may leave you only the edge of the bed to occupy as she raises that top leg upward. Don't argue with her; try to adjust yourself to her position, not vice versa.

LEGS-APART (BUTTERFLY) EXERCISE

In anticipation of this event a daily exercise is suggested for your wife to strengthen the "abductor" or legs-apart muscles. Have her lean back against a firm support with her knees together and feet flat on the floor. You place a hand on the outer surface of each of her knees and exert mild pressure to help to hold her knees together as she uses her thigh muscles to push them apart. Your hands offer the resistance necessary to tone up her abductors. Now, your biceps may be far stronger than her abductors, so don't build up your masculine ego and use so much force she can't get her thighs apart. Rather use mild resistance so that with her feet together she can gradually open her thighs to their maximum distance against your resistance. It should not take more than three seconds for her to get her legs down as far as comfortable. Take your hands off her legs as she raises them and puts her knees together and feet flat on the floor. Do this about three to ten times a day.

ACTIVE PARTICIPANT
Here we need the husband as part of the exercise itself. If you look at a bony human skeleton you will notice the wide vacant area between the upper portion of the thigh bones. In the living person this area is filled with the powerful, thick adductor muscles. These are the muscles that pull the legs together—if anyone has put a scissors hold on you in wrestling, you'll remember their power. On either male or female they are much stronger than the opposing group that pull the legs apart (abductors), which are located on the outside of the thigh bones. If a woman's legs are together or even only parallel, the abductor muscles completely close off the baby door. To get these muscles out of the way of the baby, your wife must be able to "abduct" or pull her legs apart.

BETTER PREPARED . . . EASIER PASSAGE
The better your wife can pull her thighs back and apart in the act of birth, the more room the baby has and the easier its passage is accomplished—for both the baby and the mother.

KEGEL OR PUBOCOCCYGEAL EXERCISE
You can check on your wife's progress in learning control of the muscle of the vaginal opening through which the baby actually passes by having her alternately tighten and loosen this muscle after intercourse prior to your withdrawal.

She must learn to do this exercise herself, preferably by listening to another woman describe it at your Bradley class. If no classes are available in your locality, she can learn it by analyzing the muscle action of stopping and starting urination. This is best done on arising when her bladder is full.

BLADDER INFECTIONS
Pregnant women are more prone to bladder infections so check to see if you are doing this correctly by stopping and starting urination once in a while. The rest of the time you can Kegel anywhere.

Bradley classes teach twelve weeks of progress and practice to help moms get good at this exercise. The pubococcygeus muscle is a hammock-like muscle that passes, as the name implies, from the pubic bone in front to the coccyx or tailbone in back. It is circular or sphincteric in action and serves to close off or open the three apertures in your wife's bottom: the bladder opening in front, the rectal opening in back, and the vagina between these two. The same muscle controls all three; they cannot be controlled separately.

DIFFERENCE BETWEEN TIGHTNESS AND LOOSENESS

Your wife should deliberately become consciously aware of the difference between tightness and looseness of this muscle so that she can welcome her baby with an open-door policy during the act of pushing the baby out. Like any other muscle it will become more flexible and more functional with exercise. This muscle also encourages the baby to keep its chin on its chest so that the smallest part of the head comes first. A weak muscle can make for a longer second stage and perhaps a cesarean if the baby does not keep its chin on its chest.

IMPORTANCE BEFORE AND AFTER BIRTH

There are other purposes besides proper control at the actual moment of birth. The abdominal muscles are stretched carrying the baby, and this Kegel muscle is stretched having the baby. It is important after the pregnancy and birth that these two sets of muscles be actively exercised to draw them back to their original shape and ability to function.

For years we have fussed at women to do abdominal exercises to draw their waistlines in after the pregnancy is over. It is obvious from a block away if they don't. The Kegel muscle is not so obvious but every bit as important, if not more so, as it is involved in bladder and rectal continence or control in the postpartum.

NATURAL CHILDBIRTH DIFFERENT FROM UNATTENDED

Many people confuse natural childbirth with unattended (and therefore unmedicated!) childbirth such as grandmother had out on the farm during a blizzard when the doctor couldn't get there to "give her something." She had unattended childbirth, not what we are dealing with here. The only similarity is that both lack medication, but there's a whale of a difference between the two! Grandmother was not taught muscle control, for instance.

After several unattended births without any program of muscle conditioning before, during, or after, she frequently developed inability to control her urine, especially with a full bladder, upon coughing, sneezing, lifting, etc. This also may have altered rectal control. If you don't believe this, have your wife ask her! The second reason for keeping this muscle in good flexible condition by regular exercise during pregnancy is to better its ability to return to normal function after your wife has babies.

REGULAR EXERCISING

During pregnancy our childbirth educators encourage our patients at class to exercise this muscle regularly and daily during periods of physical inactivity—e.g., while reading, sewing, watching TV. One clever teacher practices and suggests exercising the Kegel muscle while driving a car—during the periods you are stopped at a red traffic light and waiting for it to change. She also suggests to the group to exercise it at parties when the conversation is boring. This is one natural-childbirth exercise your wife can do in public, nobody will notice!

MAINTAINING VAGINAL ORGASMS

The third reason for maintaining proper tone of this muscle is that it seems to be important in maintaining the ability to achieve vaginal orgasms. Postpartum frigidity problems in some instances are related to loss of sensation due to the weakened condition of this important muscle.

RELAXATION PRACTICE

This is our final exercise and you play an important role. There are many other exercises your wife will learn at class, or from books—e.g., how to rise, lift, get to the top shelf in reaching, vertical pelvic rocking, and so on. She should adapt each one to her daily activities. If she has impaired circulation in her legs from heredity, previous poor habits, or whatever, there are special exercises in addition to cover this; these she can do without your help.

PRACTICED TO BE PERFECTED

As I said, relaxation is hardly an exercise—it's more like non-exercise—but must be practiced to be perfected, like all physical acts. As you have read in previous chapters, it is impossible to relax the body without simultaneously relaxing the mind. Here you as a coach can achieve results where none other can. We have been unable to find a coach comparable to a husband, whose familiar pattern of action is essential to mental disassociation and physical relaxation by his wife, during the intermittent pulling sensations of uterine contractions in first-stage labor. In careful anticipation of this you should establish your own pattern of verbal suggestion in short periods of concentrated relaxation, at home daily during the course of pregnancy.

ANYTIME
It could be done anytime, but perhaps the best time is when the daily chores are done, the other children are in bed, the cat has been put out, the outside doors locked, the lights turned off. In other words, you and your wife should not be distracted by thinking of anything left undone. She should be able to drift off to sleep lulled by the sound of your voice. First-stage labor is sleep imitation and the time to rehearse it is in bed just before going to sleep. Don't disrupt the program by either of you having to get up and finish something else.

PELVIC ROCK FIRST
Of course she should do her pelvic rocking first. We suggest having a soft throw rug next to the bed so her knees won't be uncomfortable. After pelvic rocking she should curl up on her side, top leg raised (with or without a pillow support—whichever she prefers) and snuggle down into her chosen favorite position for

sleep—make her "nest." Your task now is to massage her lower back area. These nightly back rubs will endear you to her—they make her feel so good.

The uterine muscle is attached in the area of the hollow of her back, the saddle area. Have skin lotion to lubricate your hands to avoid friction. Use the heel of your hand in a rotary rhythmical motion with fairly firm steady pressure. Let her suggest the details of how and exactly where to rub.

After the back rub combine verbal and touch suggestions of relaxation by whatever combination you two find effective. This varies considerably with every couple, so work out your own. Some wives like to have their husbands hum to them while relaxing; others' hair would stand on end in tension if their husband hummed. Your wife may like familiar repetitive love talk that would be utter nonsense to an outsider but gives her a feeling of security and "he loves me" reassurance. As you start this verbalization give her the reminder, "When your uterus contracts this is what we'll do."

INDICATE TENSION AREAS

Simultaneously by direct light touch suggest areas of relaxation, progressively, starting with face muscles, lips, neck, shoulders, arms, hips, legs, feet. Place one hand lightly resting on her abdomen. Her breathing should be peaceful, deep-sighing sleep breaths performed rhythmically.

NARRATIVE-FORM OF TALKING

Some mothers like to have narrative-form talking during the relaxation, describing some previous happy shared trip—"Remember when . . ." This probably relates to deep subconscious security feelings from being read to or being told stories at bedtime in early childhood and is quite useful with some mothers. Work out your own individual pattern and then repeat it each night. Repetition helps. Remind her, "After the nurse is through in the hospital, here's what we're going to do, you and I, when your uterus is working." As she gets drowsy and drops off to sleep, join her—and pleasant dreams of parenthood to you both.

PHYSICAL, MENTAL, AND EMOTIONAL RELAXATION

Physical relaxation includes touching, stroking, and rubbing. These are physical types of relaxation and you can practice these as described in this book or Bradley classes. Letting go of every muscle in the body and letting the uterus do its work is physical relaxation.

Mental relaxation involves what this mother is thinking about. Perhaps somewhere the two of you have been, seen, or done that you found to be relaxing. A beautiful image of some kind, like a rainbow or mountain scene may be useful.

Emotional relaxation is harder. It is about your wife feeling safe, secure, knowing that you are there and everything will be all right when she is concentrating on the work of labor.

Like an athletic event, preparation makes a difference.

HOW TO LIVE WITH A PREGNANT WIFE

A pregnant woman is a changed and ever-changing woman. Not only does she gradually look different, but she feels different and acts differently. Since the mind cannot be separated from the body, the physiological changes in her body affect her mind in certain subtle ways. As her constant companion, you should know and understand these ways and adjust your way of thinking and acting accordingly. Your job is more than just planting the seed. You must now tenderly nurture it, cultivate it properly, and not let weeds of anxiety, self-doubts, or unresolved hostilities spring up. Pregnant women, coached by natural-childbirth-oriented husbands, sparkle with the joy of life. The little nuisances of physical discomfort from their enlarging abdomens are jovially taken in stride as necessary nuisances without becoming all-encompassing.

CHANGES

What changes can you expect in your wife and what is your role in them?

NOT DELICATE CONDITION

First and foremost, she is not in a "delicate condition" when pregnant. She does not have to discontinue all the activities she found pleasure in before becoming pregnant. She does tire more readily and cannot accomplish as much, but she can still do the same type of things. Growing a baby in the uterus takes energy from her reserve supply. She can't bowl as many games or swim as many laps in the pool as she did before. She can bowl and she can swim when pregnant, and she should be allowed to participate in practically anything physical that she could do before. There are a few exceptions—she should not jog, jump on trampolines, jump rope, or do high diving. The first ones make the baby drop too low in the pelvis and the last one is risky due to impaired balance. Use common sense.

FALLING DOWN . . . NOT LIKELY TO HURT THE BABY

Dismiss from your mind the idea that if your pregnant wife fell down during skating, skiing, or whatever, that she would hurt her baby. Of course if she doesn't know how to fall correctly she can hurt herself—just as she could when she's not pregnant. In my career I have never known a mother to have harmed a baby by any external trauma. I suppose it is possible, but I haven't seen it. The salt water in which the baby is floating equalizes local pressure.

This idea of falling down and thereby losing a baby is a superstition that probably began with the movie *Gone with the Wind*. Rhett Butler gave his wife a shove at the top of the stairs. She gracefully tumbled down the stairs and conveniently (for the plot) had a miscarriage at the foot of the stairs. Immediately thereafter doctors' offices and hospital emergency rooms were mobbed with out-of-wedlock pregnant women who were battered black-and-blue and sore but still very much pregnant! It won't work.

SWIMMING

If your wife loves swimming, encourage her to swim anytime during her pregnancy. Swimming is an ideal exercise for pregnant women for many reasons. Suspended in water in any position, except flat on her back, her uterus is deflected upward and out. Also, expert swimmers are ideal natural-childbirth performers in labor.

"PAINLESS CHILDBIRTH"

The first patient in our series to label the method "painless childbirth" was a swimming instructor. She made me look foolish when I brought in some medical students and doctors who wanted to learn the techniques of coaching a woman in labor. I was going to check her over during first-stage labor and correct her errors. We never expect any woman to be perfect the first time in labor. I hadn't checked this mother yet, so I expected, as usual, to give directions and coach. This turned out to be one of the few times when the instructor couldn't open his mouth. There wasn't anything to correct! She had been propped up in the contour chair by her husband, who was perched on the end of the bed. He had drawn the bed tray across the space between her abdomen and thighs and they were calmly engrossed in playing cards.

I announced that with her next contraction I would check on her and correct her errors for the benefit of the medical observers. She smiled cooperatively, and when the next contraction began she said, "Excuse me a minute," to her husband, laid her hand of cards down on the tray, settled back with her arms on the supporting pillows, closed her eyes, and began the most perfect wave of total relaxation I have ever seen—reflected first in her face, then her neck, and on downward. Her breathing was perfect, deep automatic abdominal, or diaphragmatic. The more I checked, the more obvious it was that I couldn't offer a word of advice; she was perfect!

In bewilderment I asked, when the contraction was over and she had picked up her hand to resume playing, how come she was so perfect. She laughed at my puzzled face and mischievously said, "Why, Doctor, I've been teaching this myself for seven years. There's nothing to it!" I looked even more bewildered and blurted out, "You've been teaching natural childbirth?" She said, "Well, not by that name, but it's the same thing. I'm a swimming instructor and this is the same thing as floating in water!"

I had never before thought of this similarity. My pupils have taught their teacher many times since. What does one do in water to float? Relax completely, breathe gently from your abdomen, leave your eyes closed, lips parted, and breathe through your mouth. She was right. Could the fatal accidents to good swimmers who develop a leg cramp be related to inability to relax totally? You should have seen her hold her breath in second stage as she joyfully pushed into the world a healthy eight-pound baby.

Your wife doesn't have to be a swimmer to have a baby by natural childbirth. As the psychiatrist said, "You don't have to be crazy to be a psychiatrist, but it sure helps."

No, your pregnant wife is not in a delicate condition. Once a week we beg you to date her and participate in the same activities you two shared when she was not pregnant. If she gets tired, it's a good healthy physical tiredness; it won't hurt her. She will want to rest sooner. So rest. The tiredness most women complain of at the end of the day is not good physical exhaustion that follows doing something fun and physical, accompanied by deep full breathing. Sitting at a desk, housework, studying, things she feels she has to do, do not count. Try getting out to swim or bowl or dance. There is a difference.

EDUCATED

Also our problem today is different from Grandmother's day because of higher levels of education. Today wives and husbands are equally well educated; in fact, plenty of times it is the wives who have the higher education. If their only contact during the day is with their small children, they are bound to feel frustrated. Have you ever tried to carry on an intellectually stimulating conversation with small children?

LISTEN AND BE THERE FOR HER

When the two of you get home at night, whether she works away from home or not, remember she is tired also. Don't be an unthinking husband. Don't just sit in silence and eat dinner, watch TV until you get sleepy, grunt, and go to bed. How many jittery, nervous women have wailed tearfully, "If he would only talk to me"? Have some intellectual pursuits in common with your wife—have something stimulating to tell her about your day's activities. She needs to talk and be talked to.

TRAVEL

Let's dispose of another widespread misconception—that pregnant women mustn't travel. This ancient superstition dates back to the horse-and-buggy days; the springs in those buggies were not comparable to present-day cars. I sincerely doubt that even the jouncing of the buggy ever made a mother miscarry. She would have miscarried anyway.

We do advise that traveling a long distance should not be done in the last few weeks before the due date. It also should not be done at any other time of pregnancy if there is vaginal bleeding or cramping. Why? For the simple reason it's deucedly unhandy to have a miscarriage or a baby out on the highway, miles away from medical care. God only knows when your wife is going to have a baby. That assigned calendar date is utterly meaningless except as a rough guess. I've never met a baby who could read a calendar. Stay home or nearby in the last few weeks. Most babies do come after their due dates, but as sure as you plan it that way, yours will come early. Highway patrolmen are not eager to act as obstetricians.

DUE DATES

A word about due dates. Dr. Franz Carl Naegele made the rule doctors use to calculate due dates. He assumed that pregnancy lasted ten lunar months (or forty weeks). Dr. Naegele died in 1851. It wasn't until 1990, at Harvard University, that scientists checked his premise. Turns out the median length is forty-one and one-seventh weeks, not forty weeks. He was off by eight days! The actual due date is represented by a bell curve, you may have a normal full-term baby days or weeks either side of that assigned date. But the average mom, if not induced, goes eight days longer than the medical model predicts (R. Mittendorf, et al., "The Length of Uncomplicated Human Gestation," *Obstetrics & Gynecology,* volume 75, number 6, page 929, June 1990).

Prior to the last few weeks, if your wife is not bleeding or cramping (threatening to miscarry), it is perfectly all right to travel if you'll just observe a few rules of common sense. She should sleep eight or more hours out of each twenty-four. Don't overtire your wife by frantically driving night and day to get somewhere in a big hurry. Start earlier, stop and rest regularly—in a motel or hotel and a real bed—without this silly business of trying to sleep in the car. Take along a sack of her favorite fruit to nibble on while riding.

BABY FEEDS ALL THE TIME

A baby doesn't ask when dinner is ready, but depletes its mother's blood sugar by snacking all the time. So should she, on fresh fruit preferably. If her blood sugar gets low, that pregnant stomach may get motion sickness.

If your purpose in traveling is just to get there, not to see the scenery en route, it is preferable to travel by air. (Planes without pressurized cabins are not to be used at high altitude.)

Even autos with the best shock absorbers bob up and down at

high speeds and the heavy uterus is gradually tamped down and deeper into your wife's pelvis. She might, therefore, wear casual loose-fitting garments so she can sprawl on the seat, with one or both legs tucked up and under her. Make frequent stops to allow her to walk around a bit to relieve pressure discomforts, and to visit the restroom. She should ride in the front seat. She may feel more comfortable driving. That way she'll know when the curves are coming and by expecting them, compensate for them. The sudden unexpected sway makes queasy stomachs. If she likes to travel, then observing these simple rules will make it more enjoyable for her.

BATHS

Another misconception of pregnancy is that women can't take baths, or at least not in late pregnancy. I can't think of anything more miserable than a woman who can't bathe. Of all the times on earth when she needs a bath it is when she's pregnant. Extra mucus, extra perspiration, extra-tired muscles—a leisurely warm bath treats them all and should be a regular evening ritual, just before retiring, all the way through pregnancy. Heat is a wonderful physical agent to promote relaxation and restore muscles tired from carrying a baby around all day. Now, don't get carried away with overly hot baths. Keep the water body temperature or below. Hyperthermia (overheating) of the mother's body is not good for the baby.

BATHWATER DOES NOT ENTER VAGINA

The old concept that bathwater enters the vagina has been disproved. It was thought this might cause infection in the uterus in the late months of pregnancy as the cervix gradually opens a little after "false labor" contractions appear, anytime in the last three months.

This folk philosophy was shown to be wrong in two ways. First, women ignored the admonition not to bathe; they bathed anyway and got along fine without evidence of infection. Second, an enterprising doctor, recognizing this, cleverly tested to see if bathwater entered a pregnant woman's vagina. He soaked cotton vaginal tampons in a starch solution, dried them, had the mother insert and wear them each time she bathed. To her bathwater she added a few drops of iodine on each occasion.

If the water entered the vagina the starch-permeated tampons would turn blue. They didn't, so your wife can bathe all through pregnancy. She'll be a lot easier to live with.

SEX

While we're chasing away ghosts of yesterday let's chase away another one that definitely affects you. The same old concept against bathing was applied to sexual intercourse, which went: "Abstain totally in the last months of pregnancy." Comment: "Hogwash!" This was again based on an old assumption that uterine infection would result. On the surface it sounds reasonable, but in actuality there's one thing wrong with the assumption—it just isn't so!

As long as neither partner has AIDS, or a sexually transmitted disease, sex is safer without a condom. Semen contains antibiotics that kill germs, preventing infections. It also contains prostaglandins that soften the cervix, helping mothers go into labor on time and have an easier labor. The sexual climax causes contractions that tone and strengthen the uterus so that it can push when the time comes.

PROTECTED BY THE UTERUS AND BAG OF WATERS

Babies are protected from physical damage during intercourse by the uterus and the bag of waters.

Pregnant Navy wives whose husbands were at sea had no fewer infections than Air Force wives whose husbands were very much with them and who, upon careful questioning, had intercourse regularly all the way through pregnancy.

Now, here again, be sensible. We do recommend continuing relations throughout normal pregnancy—what a lovely time to make love; you don't have to worry about her getting pregnant. However, there are a few don'ts.

ON TOP . . . NOT IN LATER MONTHS

Don't lie on top of her, especially in the later months. Remember the bowling ball comparison? She's uncomfortable on her back.

Practically any position except this is all right in pregnancy. You're on your own otherwise. Let your wife decide which she finds comfortable. She should control the angle and depth of penetration. Don't argue with her! Positions mean very little to a man, but very much to a woman. A bit of further advice: be gentle. The vaginal flesh is puffy and sensitive during pregnancy from the circulation changes.

RESPONSIVENESS VARIES DURING PREGNANCY

Also, responsiveness varies. Some women enjoy increased sexual activity but some women do not particularly enjoy intercourse during pregnancy. Do not get your male ego hurt if she is not as responsive as she used to be. Physical tiredness may be affecting her, too. Be patient. She will be a responsive partner again after pregnancy is over. The increased sensitivity of the vaginal and labial flesh sometimes makes some women more responsive during pregnancy. Don't make an issue of it either way. Also, the same woman may react differently during different pregnancies.

UTERINE CRAMPS OR LABOR-LIKE CONTRACTIONS

Your wife may notice uterine cramps or increased labor-like contractions of the uterus after intercourse. Don't let her be alarmed by these; they are perfectly normal. In fact they are probably beneficial and by stimulating the uterus serve to help soften and make flexible the cervix so it will dilate more effectively during labor. If threatened miscarriage is a problem, of course abstain from intercourse and report it to your doctor.

SEX MAY AID IN LABOR

It is reported of an aboriginal tribe that men help their wives out in labor, if the contractions become ineffectual and weak, by having intercourse. I haven't yet found a cooperating hospital in which to try to do this experimentally. So far all we have achieved is the husband's presence!

Warning: The bag of waters should be intact if intercourse is tried during labor; check with your health-care professionals.

OTHER OLD WIVES' TALES

If any other old wives' tales have reached your wife's ear and bother her, by all means talk them over with your Bradley teacher and your doctor. Volumes have been written on the silly superstitions accumulated in folklore about pregnancy. The cord does not wrap around the baby's head if the wife reaches up. If your wife likes to paint, make sure to have lots of good ventilation.

Now, there are various nuisances of pregnancy that you should be acquainted with if you're going to learn to live with this ever-changing female. For convenience let's divide them into three separate groups of three months each, representing the three trimesters of pregnancy.

FIRST TRIMESTER

PRESSURE

Your wife cannot carry a steadily enlarging abdomen without feeling it. These pressure pains are more prominent in the first three months because the uterus is still small enough to sag down deeply into the bony ring of the pelvis. This is like a cork that is too small for the ring of the bottle mouth and falls into the bottle. As the uterus descends it applies pressure, in the front, to the bladder. This limits the capacity of the bladder and at the same time there is increased urine volume from the baby (your wife literally urinates for two). If you have trouble locating your wife, just stand by the bathroom door. In a few minutes she'll be either coming or going.

ROUND LIGAMENTS

There are little guy ropes attached to each upper side area of the uterus called "round ligaments." They pass from the upper side areas of the uterus into a canal on each side of the abdomen. These canals are identical to the ones through which the male spermatic tubes pass. These ligaments pass down to attachments in the major lips of the vagina, on each side. As the uterus descends it causes these structures to knuckle or bend, which produces a muscle spasm in this area. You may be walking down the street with your wife when she suddenly lets out a yelp, bends over, and holds her side. This is usually the right side (the large bowel occupies the left side of the pelvic ring and displaces the pregnant uterus more to the right), although it could be either side.

Don't try to make her keep walking, but steer her over to a shop window and have her bend down to act very interested in something in the window. After a few moments the round-ligament spasm will let up and she can comfortably walk erect again. If she has these at home, a bit of pelvic rocking followed by tailor sitting or lying on her side will relieve it. They are not a sign of something wrong, but only a result of walking on the hind legs, when these round ligaments were designed for the all-fours position. Of course, if severe side pain persists she should contact her doctor.

CONSTIPATION

In back of the descending uterus is the rectum, and the pressure from constipation can be a nuisance in early pregnancy. The proper treatment is twofold: she should get off her feet more, in the approved exercise way (pelvic rocking), to make the uterus come upward and forward, and, second, she needs to drink plenty of water and eat roughage (fresh fruit and vegetables) to keep her bowel contents soft.

SWOLLEN ANKLES AND DISTENSION OF VEINS

To each side of the pelvis are the large blood vessels of the nerves that go to the legs. Your wife may get some degree of swelling of her ankles and distension of veins of the legs, particularly if she is employed. Encourage her to do her exercises and get off her feet regularly at home. Pressure on these nerves results in odd numb or hot sensations running down her hips to her legs. They are transitory and usually come from sitting in one position too long. Remind her to move around more.

She will have a general feeling of fullness in her lower abdomen that becomes a dragging sensation if she doesn't get off her feet at regular intervals.

CIRCULATION CHANGES

As your wife's pregnancy progresses she gradually has more blood circulating through her body, estimated at one-third more volume. The veins become more noticeable, larger and bluer, especially when they are near the surface, as in the chest, legs, and hands. Incident to the increased circulation she will have increased secretion from practically every gland in her body.

INCREASED SECRETIONS

This includes the mucous glands, not only of the vagina but of the nose and mouth. She will have more saliva, more perspiration, more congestion in her sinuses. Another gland that increases its output is the thyroid gland in the throat. Your wife may get a feeling of fullness in her throat. She also absorbs extra thyroid secretions from her baby's circulation, which results in more thyroid than usual. What are the effects of extra thyroid?

She may feel warm when you and others in the room are cool. She may have palpitations of her heart, which is beating stronger anyway to push extra blood around.

HEAVY SENSATION IN HER CHEST

She may sit up suddenly in the middle of the night with a heavy sensation in her chest and throat from nervous spasm. This, coupled with palpitation of her heart, may frighten her into thinking she's having a heart attack. Reassure her, remind her to walk around a bit, and if the weather is decent, go to an open window for some big, deep, slow breaths. The feeling will pass. She may have numbness and tingling in her hands as if they are "going to sleep." Reassure her that this is to be expected. Let your medical team know of any concerns.

HER HORMONES AND FROM PLACENTA

She is receiving more hormones from her own glands and, in addition, from the donations of the placenta. As a combined result her nerves are on edge; she will be jumpy and high-strung. If you're one of the practical-joker type husbands and should sneak up behind her and surprise her, in the nonpregnant state she would smile and say, "Don't be so silly." If you tried the same trick in the pregnant state, two things would happen: (1) you'd have to get her down off the chandelier, and (2) you would hear new names for yourself that your mother never thought of.

HIGHS AND LOWS

These periods of excitability alternate with periods of depression—for no particular reason except that she's pregnant. You may come upon her unexpectedly and find her crying. Don't get too insistent about finding out exactly what's wrong. It's pretty hard for her to tell you, for the simple reason she doesn't know anything specific that's wrong! She's pregnant and she just feels like crying and to her that's a good enough reason. Darn those logical men!

LAUGH WITH . . .

Laugh *with* her but never *at* her in pregnancy, or she'll bite your head off. Her sense of humor may be depleted in pregnancy or sometimes completely warped. She will get her feelings hurt over something you thought was funny or go into peals of hysterical laughter over something you don't consider funny at all. Don't try to understand her sense of humor, just love her and make her feel how glad you are to have her—even if she does act a little nutty occasionally. The feminists criticize my use of this word, "nutty," but if they were honest, as many of my patients have commented, they would have to agree it is true.

PUFFINESS

The increased circulation, combined with a tendency for retention of salt in the body, results in a generalized puffiness of her body. This is more manifest in some areas that are rich in blood vessels—for instance, her gums. She may get sensitive gums and a pink toothbrush. She should use a less stiff brush during pregnancy and floss frequently. Her nasal mucosa is puffy and fragile and the tiny distended veins may break if she blows her nose too hard. Or she may see specks of blood in her saliva, drained from the back of her nose, especially in association with a cold. She should avoid blowing her nose whenever possible and, if she must, always blow gently with both nostrils open.

HAIR AND SKIN CARE

Her hair may lose its luster and tend to come out more when she combs it. We used to advise pregnant women not to spend a lot of money on expensive permanents, but wait until the pregnancy is over, as the hair consistency is more brittle during pregnancy. Her fingernails may peel or break more easily. Her skin will become quite dry, and she should bathe regularly with some bath oil preparation.

EYES

Her eyes are puffy and swollen internally as well as externally. She may get blurring of vision and have trouble focusing while reading. This will leave after pregnancy and does not necessarily mean she needs refraction correction.

FINGER SWELLING

Her fingers may swell, and if her rings begin to get snug she'd better remove them. If she tries to do fine sewing, she may have trouble due to stiffness of her finger joints. All of this is perfectly normal and related to an increase in her blood volume.

SKIN

There are three very important areas of her skin, important in the sense that they change during pregnancy and must be made flexible to allow stretching. From above downward they are: first, her breasts and nipples, which are going to get larger and the nipple skin darker during pregnancy. On the third day or so after the baby is born the breasts are going to suddenly get quite a bit larger, as they fill with milk. In preparation for the later need to stretch, the skin may be massaged daily with any skin cream you normally use or pure medical grade lanolin, try Lansinoh. Perfumed cream isn't necessary; avoid soap because it is drying, and gentle massage may help her feel more comfortable handling her own breast.

BREAST-FEEDING

Successful breast-feeding depends upon learning how. Read *The Womanly Art of Breastfeeding* (La Leche League International,

Plume, 2004) and go to La Leche League meetings to learn how, including positioning the baby at the breast. Bradley classes also cover this and there are instructions in *The Bradley Method Student Workbook*. Positioning is very important to avoid sore nipples.

COLOSTRUM

A small amount of sticky yellow-white substance may be secreted from the nipples in the later months. It is called colostrum, is perfectly normal, and can be rubbed right back into the skin along with the moisturizer as nature's little contribution.

SKIN FLEXIBILITY

The second area of skin that must be made flexible so that it will stretch comfortably is your wife's abdomen. Moisturizer should be applied and worked into the skin daily. This prevents the surface layer of skin from cracking or itching. It does not necessarily prevent the formation of "stretch marks," which seem to be inescapable in fair-skinned mothers. These are the reddish streaks that appear on the lower abdomen, hips, and often outer aspects of the breasts during pregnancy. They will turn a silvery white months after the baby is born and should be proudly worn as "service stripes" of motherhood. Good nutrition also helps the skin. Be sure you are getting a healthy diet, with healthy fats or oils to give the skin elasticity from the inside.

SOAP

Soap is a strong alkaline agent and is an insult to human skin, as it tends to dry out natural skin oils. Regardless of the advertising claims for how mild a soap is, or how much moisturizer the manufacturer adds, plain warm water is far better, with bath oil added.

QUEASINESS

Probably the peskiest nuisance of the first trimester is the queasy feeling. This is related to constantly lowered blood sugar due to the demands of the baby upon your wife's circulating blood. Later on, her body will compensate for this new demand and release extra glycogen into the blood from liver storage quantities. The body seems slow in calling out the reserves, though, and she will be "icky" to some degree during the first three months.

By "icky" we mean light-headed, shaky, dizzy with nausea or a squeamish feeling in her stomach. If she ignores these signs and doesn't replenish her blood sugar, they can go on to a blackout feeling or even actual fainting or severe nausea with vomiting or both. The treatment is based on the baby's wanting and taking nourishment from her bloodstream continuously, day and night.

TAKES FIRST . . .

The baby is demanding in his dependency. He takes whatever he needs whenever he needs it. He doesn't ask Mama first if she can spare it. He also doesn't starve four hours and then stuff himself for a few minutes as adults are accustomed to do. As a result, there are three commandments of pregnancy regarding how to eat that you should help your wife achieve. The troublesome queasy feeling will either disappear or be reduced to a minimum.

There are wrist bands that put pressure on specific points to help with nausea and are used for seasickness. The FDA has also approved a new device that you put on your wrist to help with nausea during pregnancy. Ask your doctor or midwife if you have nausea excessively if these new devices would help.

Pregnancy Commandment One: "Thou shalt not let thy stomach go empty."

The pregnant woman should nibble (baby is little and it doesn't take much) between meals on natural sweets every hour on the hour. This need not mean she will get fat; we said nibble, not stuff. The only approved form of sweets is honey and fresh fruit, in any variety. Both have a readily absorbed and assimilated form of natural sugar that is converted to blood sugar rapidly, plus beneficial vitamins.

FRESH FRUIT

She should be a good fresh-fruit shopper and have several varieties available at all times to avoid monotony. Pick up fresh fruit for her on your way home from work, as it spoils rapidly and cannot be stocked. If she gets stuck away from home and begins to get light-headed and squeamish, and no fresh fruit is available, as a temporary expedient she'd better nibble on any form of sweets she can find. Working pregnant women should take along some fruit to nibble on intermittently between meals. Tell the employer it's doctor's orders.

I recall a schoolteacher who continued teaching while pregnant—as well she should. She took a sack of grapes along to school and furtively ate two grapes every hour. She got along fine. One morning, in a hurry, she forgot her grapes and didn't have time to go back for them. She tried to stick it out until noon but didn't make it. She got light-headed around ten a.m., vomited at eleven a.m., and fainted at eleven-thirty a.m.

LOWER BLOOD PRESSURE

Most women routinely carry a lower blood pressure than men. Why, I don't know. I have various theories about it, but my wife doesn't seem to agree with any of them. Low average blood pressure means longevity (women have a habit of outliving men). Those with low blood pressure should not suddenly change from a horizontal to a vertical position (it makes them dizzy), and they should nibble between meals even when not pregnant. Low blood sugar combined with low blood pressure produces a tired, irritable person. In World War II, when women invaded the factories in great numbers while their menfolk were invading the battlefields, it was found that there were fewer accidents and more productive woman-hours if they had coffee breaks between meals. The benefit wasn't so much the coffee as it was the pastries that accompanied it. Women with low blood pressure were meant to eat lightly and frequently, pregnant or not.

Dismiss from your mind and hers that her nibbling on sweets between meals, especially fresh fruit, will result in your being married to an obese woman. Overweight is more likely to result if she doesn't. Going for long hours empty makes her so frantically hungry that she tends to overeat when mealtime finally comes. An enterprising promoter made a fortune on weight pills to be taken at ten a.m. and three p.m. The pills were remolded hard candy from a leftover Christmas stock, to which he added an insignificant dab of vitamins. He had many testimonials as to their effectiveness. Remember your mother admonishing you not to eat sweets just before your dinner, as you wouldn't eat all your dinner if you did? Same principle.

Pregnancy Commandment Two: "Thou shalt not overload thy pregnant stomach."

There are several reasons for this. One, there isn't as much room. The rising uterus limits the space. Two, there is a delayed emptying time of the stomach in pregnancy from the muscle-relaxing effect of hormones. Food tends to stay there and form gas, especially foods that are slow to digest, such as cauliflower, onions, green peppers, beans, etc. This results in the "heart-burn" of pregnancy. Nothing to do with the heart, but it produces gas pressure under the ribs. Your wife should avoid foods that cause this and ask her health-care provider for antacid suggestions. Some women like papaya for this.

ROLLER-COASTER EFFECT ON BLOOD SUGAR
Thirdly, sudden high elevations of blood sugar from a lot of food at once will result in a compensatory letdown drop of blood sugar later.

DINE LEISURELY
If you and your wife go out for a dinner engagement, that's fine. You should do this regularly, since there will be plenty of times

when neither of you will feel like cooking. However, during pregnancy, take plenty of time, dine leisurely, discuss pleasant topics between courses.

Pregnancy Commandment Three: "Thou shalt not go to bed on an empty stomach—have a protein nightcap."

Grandmother's morning sickness of pregnancy has changed since we began insisting on a bedtime snack of protein. Morning sickness was an inescapable result of too-long emptiness. Grandmother ate supper at five p.m., then didn't eat again until about six a.m.—thirteen hours between meals is too long.

PROTEIN

The reason for protein food is that it takes longer to convert to blood sugar and the effect lasts longer during the sleeping hours. Your wife should choose the protein she likes best—leftover lean meat, hard-boiled egg, cheese sandwich on whole-wheat bread, high-protein breakfast cereal, yogurt, etc. Again, it doesn't take much, but it takes some.

NIBBLE AT NIGHT

If your wife gets up to go to the bathroom during the night, and she will, it's a good idea for her to nibble on a little something out of the refrigerator before returning to bed. This helps tide her over until morning. Actually snacking often helps morning sickness all day long. It may not eliminate it—but it sure helps. Keep something beside your bed to eat upon awakening, before she sits up, or actually gets up.

NUTRITION DURING PREGNANCY

Your wife may get bizarre cravings for some ungodly food at some ungodly hour. Quit grumbling, get dressed, and go get it! Some pregnancies don't manifest these odd cravings, but, then again, some do. No one knows why; it's just part of the general picture. Make a joke out of it—laugh, don't act misused. After all, you helped to start all this business in the first place.

NUTRITION NEEDS PLANNING

Good nutrition starts with planning. Whoever selects and prepares the meals should be well versed in what constitutes good nutrition for pregnant women. If you share this job, both of you should be well informed on selection and preparation of foods.

Today there are many fads and folktales and you need a basic idea of what is involved. First and foremost, regardless of her body weight, she should never go on a low-calorie or starvation diet. She is pregnant and the baby needs food, especially protein, even if she thinks she doesn't. She should be restrictive not in the quantity of food but in the quality. She should eat all the protein (lean meat, eggs, milk, cheese, whole-grain cereal) her appetite calls for. The baby needs protein to grow on. If she has a weight problem and tends to gain excessive weight, help her by being aware of her nutritional choices.

SALT

All women get some degree of edema, or water retention, when pregnant. In the bygone days, women were put on low-calorie as well as low-salt diets to counteract this weight gain. Today we know this is not good; women should always have adequate high protein in their diets to protect them from toxemia and to give proper nutrition to their babies (T. H. Brewer, *Metabolic Toxemia of Late Pregnancy, A Disease of Malnutrition*. Academy Publications, 2004). Protein and fluid intake are crucial; it is important to salt your food to taste.

DIURETICS

Diuretics, or "water pills," are to be condemned, as crossing the placenta, as most things do, they have a deleterious effect on the baby. A good reference book is *What Every Pregnant Woman Should Know: The Truth About Diet and Drugs in Pregnancy*, by Gail Brewer with Tom Brewer, M.D. (New York: Penguin, 1985).

ANIMAL FATS AND OILS

Some fat is essential, but keep it to a moderate level. Broil that meat instead of frying it. Eat the lean part instead of the fat.

Fresh vegetables, tossed salads—all she wants, but try vinegar, lemon juice, or non-oily salad dressing, or mixtures of these, instead of the ordinary mayonnaise salad dressings.

MILK
Some women connect milk with motherhood and guzzle a gallon a day. Four cups are plenty. I have seen women who abhor milk hold their noses and choke it down because they were pregnant. This is ridiculous. However, your wife should drink milk if she likes it, since it is an excellent (and cheap!) source of protein and calcium. If you're lactose-intolerant, you can choose other high-protein, high-calcium foods.

WHITE FLOUR IN ITS VARIOUS FORMS
The brown outer kernel of the wheat seed is taken off and given to cattle in the form of bran and "shorts." The white inner portion, consisting mostly of starch and a small amount of protein, is ground up to make flour for people because it's prettier. We tend to have healthy cattle and unhealthy people as a result. There are many good whole-wheat products in the supermarket. Read labels.

Careful shopping in pregnancy is very important. When others are eating pastry products between meals, she should be nibbling on fresh fruit instead.

SUGAR IN ITS VARIOUS FORMS
Candy, canned fruit, pastry goods, etc., seem to produce an obsession for more, and more, and more. It's deucedly hard to eat just one piece of candy, or just one little sweet roll, or just one piece of bread and jelly. Craving sweets may also indicate a need for protein.

HONEY
Bees come to our rescue here with their sweet concoction, honey. Chemists have yet to analyze all its contents, but in general, it is used to raise the blood sugar of athletes (swimmers, boxers, etc.) to give them additional energy rapidly. Pregnant women also

need additional energy. It is not a matter of calories, but of efficient and immediate utilization to produce energy that prompts us to suggest honey as a substitute, whenever possible, for the sugar bowl. Also, for reasons I don't understand, it does not produce that obsession for more, and more, and more. In fact, honey will produce nausea if overused, so it is easy to limit its use.

SECOND TRIMESTER

As your wife enters the fourth month of pregnancy you may note a change of personality. She looks better. She becomes radiant. She sparkles and is fun to be around. This second three-month period is the most comfortable part of pregnancy. Why?

ACCLIMATION PERIOD (GETTING USED TO)

Many reasons. The queasy feeling is rare because her body is adjusting to pregnancy. The uterus has grown large enough so that it doesn't fit in the pelvic ring anymore and now is deflected forward instead of downward. This produces the little O or bulge in her tummy that is external evidence of fertility now, and a convenient place to rest her book while reading. The pressure pains described in the first trimester have let up. She still gets an occasional round-ligament cramp in her sides, but the pressure is less on all those organs deep in the pelvis. Her personality reflects happiness. We doctors notice it on office calls. Instead of that long list of "what the heck's going on inside me" type of complaints she meets us with a cheery greeting.

BELLY BUTTON

The navel will now gradually begin to protrude instead of being inverted. Her breasts are enlarging and were never more lovely. She should be proud of her figure and she may need an adjustable maternity or nursing bra now.

MOVEMENT OF BABY

Anywhere from the fourth to fifth month she will feel the movement of her baby for the first time. Up to then she has suspected that the rumor she was pregnant was probably true, but this is different! She knows she is pregnant now; she can feel the baby kick! It's a delightful feeling to a mother; the wonderment of the miracle of life will occupy her even more.

BABY KICK PLUS FIVE MONTHS

There is an old rule of thumb that if you add five months to the date she first felt your baby kick it will be the true or more accurate due date. This, the first baby movement, is hard to assess, as the early movements are momentary and she will not be really sure. Then, later on, after it is kicking regularly, she will conclude, why, that must have been it last week. Just for fun, arrive at a date when she felt the first real thump (not the flutter that precedes it), add five months, and see what you come out with.

This supposedly takes into consideration the rate of growth of the individual baby. If it's a speedball in growth and kicks early, it should come early. If it's a slowpoke in growth and kicks its mother late, it should come late. Maybe! There are too many variables involved to be dependable—and even current technology has failed to accurately predict due dates. The variables include estimating how much salt water is enclosing this particular child, its position in the uterus, etc. But it keeps up your interest. You can make up a "pool" with your wife, relatives, and friends—as you do with World Series scores—and see who wins. I've seen a lot of excitement from a husband in the birthing room over winning the pool.

BABY HICCUPS

You or your wife may notice at times a slow, rhythmical little jumping motion of her abdomen. It is too slow to be a heartbeat, too regular to be arms or legs moving. What is the baby doing? We've heard that question many times. The baby is hiccupping. Babies swallow the salt water they are immersed in and occasionally, just as on the outside, they get hiccups.

Your wife is no invalid nor in any delicate condition. Spend time together and have fun. Now is the time to do the shopping for the baby supplies and plans for his or her reception. Help plan and choose the colors or paint the crib and get things ready. After all, it's your baby, too, so take an interest.

Charge her storage battery of love. Mother love to a baby has been defined as the gradual release of husband love and affection that was built up and stored from attentions received during pregnancy. Don't get nauseating about it, but give her little extras. Tell her how much you love her and show her how much—she never gets tired of being reminded.

DATE NIGHT(S)

Let's add a husband commandment here: date your wife at least once a week. Do the things with her you found joy in sharing before you were married. Why did you pick her as your choice of companion for life? Don't quit living just because somebody put your names on a piece of paper headed "marriage certificate." If you have other children, get a babysitter on this once-a-week occasion. Don't say you can't afford this. There are no reasonable excuses. You can trade around and take turns babysitting with another young couple in a similar situation. Money helps, I'll grant you, but what inexpensive things did you do that were fun before you married? Do them again.

TAKE THE TIME

And don't tell me you can't spare the time. Take the time! I don't care what sort of work you're in or how hard you're struggling to achieve some goal. First things first, and keeping those home fires burning brightly takes precedence over anything else. Many a man gets so wrapped up in his work that he forgets and neglects the other facets of his role. What does it profit you to "arrive" only to find you have lost your companion somewhere along the road? It can get mighty lonely up there.

THIRD TRIMESTER

This is the old homestretch. As your wife enters the seventh month her abdomen becomes ponderously heavy. She will have to move around more slowly now. Making the bed, which took five minutes before, now takes fifteen. Do your share of the housework and get extra help if you can. She will tire more easily now. She will still want to go places, but she won't want to do as much and she'll want to come home earlier. Why? The uterus is larger and heavier and harder to carry around. The presenting part of the baby, that part that is coming out first (usually the head), is being pushed down into the pelvic ring by the forces of the uterine muscle contracting. It contracts at irregular intervals for irregular durations—this is called false labor, pre-labor, or medically, Braxton Hicks contractions. Such muscular action could be compared to that of a player who after sitting idly on the bench starts warming up in expectation of playing in the game soon. He would run up and down the sidelines, flexing his playing muscles, getting them ready.

WARMING UP

Your wife's uterus is now doing the same thing—warming up. The football player does not act with as much vigor on the sidelines as he will after entering the game. Similarly, your wife's uterus does not contract as hard, or as long, or as often as it will "later in the game." It contracts hard enough, though, to put pressure on her lower back and tailbone. It brings back the bladder pressure, rectal pressure, leg swelling, vein swelling, and so forth, described in detail in the first trimester.

REST, PREPARE

She should get off her feet more. She should rest more. She should do horizontal pelvic rocking now four times a day, at midmorning (ten a.m.), after lunch at midday, again at midafternoon (three p.m.), and, of course, at night before retiring. After each pelvic rocking session, she should lie down for at least ten minutes (longer if she wishes) on her side with her top leg drawn up. She should sit or lie down ten minutes or more of each hour if she's at home. At work, she should seek out a ladies' lounge after lunch if she doesn't have her own office, pelvic rock, and rest a few minutes before returning to work.

She can remain active and accomplish a lot of things yet. She should not stay too long in any position, even approved ones, or she'll get stiff and uncomfortable. She will want to go out but not to formal or long drawn-out affairs. Renting a video may sound like a pretty good option.

BABY'S HEARTBEAT

One of the pleasant aspects after the seventh month is to have you, the husband, listen to the baby's heartbeat. The doctor listens to your baby's heart rate with the ultrasound Doptone, or with a fetoscope. However, don't be too impressed with his fancy gadgets, because at home you can hear the baby by just putting your ear on your wife's abdomen and pressing it steadily against the skin. The only reason the doctor doesn't listen directly is that it's rather undignified.

Get out your watch, after you have placed your ear at the proper point to hear the sound, and count the number of beats per minute. I would suggest you start your listening on the left side of her abdomen and just a little lower than her navel. Most babies lie with their backs to the left of midline, but not necessarily. If you don't hear it there, let your ear wander around until you do. What will it sound like? Like a watch ticking. The rate averages 140 beats per minute, which is often twice the rate of the mother, but the baby's rate may vary as much as from 100 to 160, more or less. There may be other sounds that confuse you—the gurgles and swishes of intestinal movements or a uterine "soufflé" sound made by the flowing of blood through the placenta. After a little practice you'll be able to distinguish which is the baby's heartbeat.

BOY OR GIRL?

Superstition has it that if the fetal heart rate is over 140, the baby will be a girl, if it is less than 140, a boy. Boys are slow and girls fast, *supposedly*. Theoretically, if the child will grow to large stature its heart needs to beat more slowly; if destined for small stature, its heart will beat faster. An elephant's heartbeat is slower than a hummingbird's.

Count the heartbeat all you want to, but don't count on the boy-girl prediction. It's all guesswork and fun—like what's in a Christmas present. But you still have to wait for Christmas Day to open the gift to see what's in it. Don't get your heart set on one or the other; you may be surprised in spite of heartbeats.

AMNIOCENTESIS

There is a way of telling whether it's a boy or girl before its birth. A doctor can insert a long needle through the abdomen and uterus and withdraw a sample of the amniotic fluid. It can be spun down in a centrifuge and the cellular patterns studied. This procedure is called amniocentesis. But who in the world wants to go through all that just to ruin the pleasant surprise of opening your presents at Christmas? All tests have a margin for error. None of them are 100 percent accurate, including ultrasound and amniocentesis. Besides, we rather hope you'll accept the baby regardless of its gender.

In the last trimester the baby is so close to your wife's rib cage that its movements may give her "pregnancy pleurisy." This is not actually pleurisy but is a sharp twinge under or along her ribs similar to pleurisy. It comes, again, from the pressure of the baby's movements. No treatment is effective except getting her off her feet more often.

HARDER TO BREATHE AND HEARTBURN

In addition, the pressure upward of the growing uterus will produce a shortness of breath in general and an occasional sudden suffocating sensation in particular. This sensation occurs when the baby straightens out its legs and suddenly interferes as the diaphragm is about to descend in inspiration. This gives the same sensation to your wife as if, just as she happened to breathe in, someone clapped their hand over her mouth. She won't really suffocate. If the breathing muscle can't descend at that moment, all she has to do is open her rib cage and chest-breathe or sigh until the baby withdraws its feet. These baby feet may also temporarily block emptying time of her stomach, and burping and heartburn are characteristic results.

DROP OR ENGAGE IN PELVIS

Somewhere along the course of the third trimester the baby will "drop," or engage itself in the pelvis. This is not as abrupt as it sounds. Rather, the baby sort of settles down at a lower level and keeps gradually getting lower, due to the effect of the downward pull from gravity and the effect of pre-labor uterine contractions. When the baby drops it does not denote that labor is due shortly, or even correlate with the onset of labor. There simply is no reliable sign that one can depend on to tell when labor will start.

ASSORTED SIZES

If babies were all born an identical size, we could then estimate on that basis. But babies insist on coming in assorted sizes. Perhaps it's just as well because we doctors can't estimate their size accurately anyway. Large, medium, and small is as close as we can come. Even with ultrasound scans we can be off by as much as four pounds or more. The passenger won't hold still and manages to elude measurement. After "dropping," the baby may put pressure on the sciatic nerve going to your wife's hip. This "sciatica of pregnancy" is normal and produces numbness and pain temporarily in her hip.

HOT FLASHES

Your wife will occasionally have "hot flashes" in this phase of pregnancy. This is not a sign of the change of life but the effect of increased blood volume, psychological factors, anxiety, malnutrition or vitamin depletion, exhaustion, or frequently the now-large uterus contracting and thereby forcing the blood from its muscles back into the mother's circulation. She feels intermittently warm and then, as the uterus relaxes and the blood runs back, momentarily clammy and chilly. This alternation of circulation generally also produces brain effects.

PANICKY FEELINGS

She may experience panicky feelings—usually manifested by sudden fears that she "can't possibly go through with it." "It" in this case, is all of motherhood—pregnancy, labor, birth, and child rearing. She gets little panicky, trapped feelings, and has doubts of her ability as a mother. Give her a gentle reminder that this feeling has been manifested similarly in all women, but they find out later, sometimes to their surprise, that they perform beautifully when the time comes and become admirable mothers.

NIGHTMARES

The same brain phenomena occurring during sleep along with increased hormones and anxiety/excitement can produce bizarre nightmares during the last three months. Your wife may awaken startled, having dreamed that she had a two-headed calf instead of a baby, or multiple babies—"They couldn't shut them off." The latter phenomenon probably is related to the conscious wondering during the day: "How can one baby have so many feet? It must be more than one." The truth is all the movement that puzzles her is not feet alone; there are hands, elbows, knees, as well as feet. With all this baby activity, now is the time to help her prepare more carefully for sleep.

We have carefully gone over the details of the nuisances of pregnancy, the little discomforts, pressure pains, etc. This was purposeful in order to acquaint you with how your wife feels during pregnancy and why. I firmly believe in the power of positive thinking, so let's wrap it up on a pleasant note.

BEST TIME OF YOUR LIVES

In spite of all these little nuisances, this procreative time can be the most pleasant part of your lives. The rest of your lives you may both look back upon these days with tenderness and a fond smile. Women often wish they could live them over again, in spite of the nuisances. I could also give you a list of several hundred sterile women, or women married to sterile men, who would cheerfully trade places with a pregnant mom. Couples even spend tens of thousands of dollars with specialists who try to manipulate nature to obtain fertilization.

They may never know the thrill and satisfaction of being part of the miracle of giving life to a new individual—one who blends the physical and mental inheritances of your respective bodies and souls. This experience will manifest forever your shared love, a new person to carry on where you must leave off, to make the world a better place. It helps to remember that while the nuisances of pregnancy are few, trivial, and finite, the blessings of parenthood are many, ennobling, and lasting.

9

"DOES MY WIFE HAVE TO BE 'CUT'
(HAVE AN EPISIOTOMY)?"

A grandmother of one of our young mothers once said to me, "I had midwives; they knew how to deliver babies without all that cuttin'!"

Grandma was right. Midwives in olden days were not allowed to "cut"; that was a doctor's privilege. I have the greatest respect for midwives, then and now. There are many excellent ones in practice today who serve a noble purpose now and in the development of birthing in this country and other countries.

However, I know there are occasions where a little cutting does a great deal of good. No, your wife doesn't have to be cut. With term-sized babies the cut is beneficial in some instances. In my old-fashioned way, I felt cutting was needed by less than about half of my patients. That was when other doctors were doing 100 percent episiotomies. Today I would do a lot fewer.

CLASSIC TECHNIQUE OPTION

To illustrate my point, I tell patients if they don't want to be cut under any circumstances we will, at their insistence, use the old midwife technique of getting a baby out that relatively small opening without cuts or tears.

What was the old midwife technique? I'm amazed to find today's childbearing generation hasn't the foggiest idea. Let's study a little history together. Perhaps you have seen movies of olden days—*Gone with the Wind*, for example. The midwife's first request, to all concerned, is for what? Hot water! Not a teacupful but buckets, tubs, pans. What does she do with all that hot water?

I have asked our prenatal classes that question and got quite a variation in answers. "It makes the husband cut wood to keep him out of the way." "It's to make tea for the doctor." No, the midwife puts salt in these steaming buckets of water, then she starts rounding up clean cloths, freshly ironed to sterilize them. She has been known to improvise with her own petticoats in time of need. The cloths are torn into strips and placed in the hot salt water to be used as steaming compresses to be applied to the laboring woman's vaginal area. After one cloth cools down a hot replacement is applied, and so on through the entire course of labor.

HOT SALTWATER COMPRESSES

These hot saltwater compresses are alternated with applications of olive oil and manual massaging of the vaginal opening to effect stretching. If you have ever soaked some minor infection of your skin in hot salt water for a time, you will recall how the skin becomes loose and wrinkled, losing its normal elasticity. This prolonged soaking combined with vigorous manual massage and stretching results in a gaping aperture.

The problem is that human flesh, unlike rubber, does not spring back into its original shape. Even the best grade of rubber never quite assumes its original proportions after stretching, and if repeatedly stretched, it becomes very flaccid eventually. The same applies to vaginas. All human flesh has a different degree of elasticity, but skin, so treated, has a tendency to remain stretched.

No, we didn't keep buckets of hot water in delivery rooms when I started out, as we felt doing the little cuts called "episiotomies" prevented overstretching of the vagina. It is true, however, that natural-childbirth physical training greatly reduces the need for large cuts, and in some more flexible flesh, any cuts. If needed, ours are done just before the baby is born, and are of the midline variety. They are far smaller than those needed for untrained patients.

Why do humans need these when animals don't? I honestly don't know. I have a pet theory, which, like most armchair philosophy, is probably wrong. I'll give it to you for what it's worth.

HUMANS DIFFER BY WALKING ERECT AND WEARING CLOTHES

The human animal differs from all others in two important respects. It walks erect and wears clothes—or at least some cover-up. Even the briefest bikini bathing suit includes a cloth covering of the vagina—on some, this is nearly all it covers! We now have "topless" bathing suits but not as yet "bottomless." In the erect-postured human animal the sun would seldom shine on the vaginal area even if it weren't clothed. (I have had the privilege of acting as obstetrician for nudists, and from the physical standpoint I could not argue with those suntanned-all-over mothers. Their skin is more flexible, less brittle.)

BRITTLE AND CHAPPED SKIN

The skin around the vagina in non-nudist mothers is usually brittle and chapped. We apply to this condition the term "panty rash," chapped lips of the vagina regularly irritated by moist cloth and the friction from movement. This is the same condition as "diaper rash" in babies and "jockstrap itch" in men who perform regularly as athletes.

MOISTURE AND MUCUS CAUSE CHAFING AND IRRITATION

In babies the source of moisture on the cloth is obvious, in men athletes it comes from perspiration, in women, particularly pregnant women, it comes from perspiration and vaginal mucus. Both are normal and profuse in pregnancy. They cause moisture in clothes too close to the skin, which results in chafing and irritation. If a wet cloth were rubbed constantly on the oral lips, they, too, would become chapped and would crack when the dentist says, "Open wide." Animals have an advantage here. Not only is their vaginal area uncovered, they are constantly exposed to the toughening and evaporating effect of sunlight, so they have vaginal skin that is flexible instead of brittle.

Enough theory. What's the practical application with your pregnant wife? If you want to clear up diaper rash on a baby, remove the diaper, the irritant. Put it on the crib mattress rather than on the baby.

PANTIES CAUSE IRRITATION

This is also true for women. If you remove the panties, the irritant, you improve the skin. Custom does not work in our favor though, men, and I wish you better luck than I've had. These flimsy garments could not possibly add much warmth, but women seem to have become accustomed to them. We do wish you would encourage your wife not to wear them at all or not to wear them around the house. Suggest that she hang them up with her purse, car keys, or coat; put them on, if she must, as she leaves, take them off as she returns. Or as a last resort, wear droopy old garments that do not fit tightly against the vaginal skin. The tight-fitting, completely covering panty hose are every bit as confining and interfering as panties. Bare bottoms are healthiest.

The internal vaginal skin is called "mucosa" and is constantly moist with mucus. This skin does not need cutting, as it unfolds quite readily when the baby descends. The vaginal mucus is normal and in constant production, although more plentifully during pregnancy, as previously mentioned. There is normally no need for douching, as washing out the mucus defeats the purpose for which it exists. Do not inject solutions up your nostrils to wash out mucus, either. You wouldn't have a clean nose if you did, but, eventually, an infected, dry, irritated one.

CLEAN AND CLEANSING

The vaginal mucus is in itself clean and cleansing in its action, from above downward. It is there for a reason and should be left alone in healthy women. I enjoy teasing two of my friends, a dentist and a throat specialist, telling them that as an obstetrician I deal with the cleanest opening of the body, whereas they deal with the one laden with bacteria. If there is any doubt about this, the study of the stained mucus smear from the respective areas will be very revealing. Normal vaginal mucus contains a single species of bacillus (Doderlein), which maintains an acid reaction that prevents the growth of other bacteria.

ABSTAIN FROM SOAP

In the care of the external skin of the vagina your wife should abstain from using soap, which tends to remove natural protective skin oils, and bathe gently without soap. After rinsing and drying gently she should then anoint this area with any unperfumed moisturizer.

If she follows these suggestions, your wife's flexible skin will need very little in the way of incisions or perhaps none. The perineum was designed for birthing.

EPISIOTOMIES

When necessary these little cuts (episiotomies) are done in the outer skin at the back corner of the vagina, in the tough flesh that is in front of the rectum. This flesh is tendonous in nature. With the oral lips, chapping is most likely to happen at the two corners of the mouth. The corners of the vaginal lips are front and back. By doing the little incision at the flexible back corner we release tension to prevent any cracks of the skin at the rigid front corner where the vaginal lips surround or house the clitoris. The clitoris is important for proper sexual function. We do not want scars, cracks, or incisions at this corner, as they may interfere with sexual response later.

PRESSURE EPISIOTOMY . . .
NO ANESTHETIC NEEDED

Even though we use no anesthetic we make a bet with our mothers that they can't tell their husbands if or when we do this little incision. We wink at the husband and show him the scissors at the time we perform it, then after the baby is born ask the mother to tell her husband just exactly with which push we did the cut. We have had to refund no fees because properly applied pressure, the natural anesthetic, is most effective. After the baby and placenta have been passed, we leisurely inject Novocain in the edges of the cut and put in the few small stitches. The Novocain is necessary then, as the pressure anesthetic is gone.

I recall teasing a doctor's wife to illustrate the effectiveness of God's anesthetic to a group of student nurses and new interns. She was an R.N. as well as a close friend and therefore eligible for teasing. In the course of pushing during second stage, I made her a bet of fifty dollars that she couldn't accurately tell the ring of observers at what moment I performed the episiotomy. She got a mischievous gleam in her eye and bet she could. I knew what she was basing her confidence on. She had had other natural-childbirth babies and she knew that you can perceive additional pressure contact at this area, not pain but pressure sensation. Being a nurse, she also knew where the scissors were kept—in a pan of sterile water nearby.

To fool her I hid an extra pair of scissors in one hand, then with each push simply touched the area, just to confuse her. On one of the pushes I used the hidden scissors, and, instead of just touching, actually did the incision. It was obvious to the observers that she could not tell any difference. On the next push I reached over into the pan, got the regular scissors, but just touched her with my gloved hand. She triumphantly informed the audience I had cut her that time, much to their delight. She lost the bet but helped to demonstrate a great fundamental natural-childbirth fact: properly applied pressure prevents pain.

Another illustration came in the form of a letter from a furious former patient. She had had several babies by natural childbirth, then moved to a distant city. She went to a new doctor who practiced natural childbirth—only he was one of those who confuse hypnotic suggestion with the physical factors of pain relief. In fact, he didn't believe there were physical factors. He obtained the history of her previous episiotomies without medication and learned that she hadn't felt them. This he interpreted as pure mental suggestion.

At the birth of the baby he performed the episiotomy at the proper time while she was pushing, but then went ahead and put in the stitches later without Novocain, insisting to her during his action that, "It is numb, it doesn't hurt." Her letter was rather vivid: "It hurt like hell!" Properly prepared hypnotic trances can produce analgesia by suggestion. With this I have no argument, but do not confuse this with the physical facts of natural childbirth. I have used both approaches and found that the simplicity of natural childbirth compared to the complexity of hypnosis is like wheeling up a cannon to shoot a sparrow when a BB gun would have sufficed.

In summary, do not build up a mighty issue over these simple little cuts. If she fell down and cut her knee in a similar way, she would go to the doctor and he would inject Novocain around the edges of the cut and hold it together with a few simple stitches. She would pay little attention to the whole thing. The cut made for having a baby is in a different location but similar in nature and management. The main difference between the two actually is that the cut on the perineum will heal remarkably faster and with far less discomfort. The extra circulation associated with pregnancy promotes more rapid healing.

TWELVE THINGS OUR MOTHERS DO
TO HELP AVOID AN EPISIOTOMY

(Remember an episiotomy is a medical procedure that may be needed occasionally but is not part of the natural process.)

1. **Good nutrition.** A well-nourished mother has healthier skin that can stretch with the process of labor.

2. **Squatting.** Squatting on a daily basis with the feet flat on the floor is the only exercise we have that helps to give elasticity to the perineum, the skin between the vagina and anus. Women who squat have a perineum that is thinner and more elastic. Those who do not squat are more likely to tear because the perineum is thicker and less likely to stretch easily.

3. **Air.** For the health of the perineum light and air are important. Perhaps one of the worst things a mother can do is wear tight-fitting clothes like panty hose. Around the house wear a long flowing skirt with no underwear or at least breathable cotton underwear.

4. **Kegel.** Daily Kegel practice throughout pregnancy helps the baby to put its chin on its chest in labor, and encourages the smallest part of the baby's head to come first. The smaller part coming first helps the perineum to stretch normally.

5. **No soap.** Soap can be drying and takes away the natural oils, causing irritation to the skin, especially the perineum. A warm bath works well without soap.

6. **Lotion and massage.** Putting lotion on the perineum can be soothing. Be sure you are using a lotion that you are not allergic to. Perineal massage is not necessary, especially the perineal massages you see on the Internet. There does not seem to be any difference in the episiotomy rate. Gentle massage as you apply the lotion is fine.

7. **Talk to your doctor or midwife in advance.** Chances are you have a doctor or midwife who is supportive of natural childbirth and probably has lots of patients. Do not assume that they can remember what everyone wants. Talk to them ahead of time so they know what you want. Make sure they are in agreement so there are no surprises.

8. **Be patient.**   Some babies pop right out in second stage, some take their sweet time. Push to the point of comfort.

9. **Keep your elbows up and out and knees back.**   During second-stage contractions, to help prevent tearing. Putting your knees apart (widening) as far as possible overstretches the perineum and makes it more likely that a tear will occur. If the doctor or midwife does need to do a small midline episiotomy it is not as likely to extend if your elbows are up and out and knees back.

10. **Push with self-control.**   When the urge to push starts, take a minute and think about how hard your body is telling you to push. Push to the point of comfort. That might be with all your might, especially in the beginning, or you may feel like a gentle push as the perineum is stretching. Tune in to your body and follow those clues.

11. **Remind the doctor or midwife about your wishes at the birth.** You may have talked to your doctor or midwife weeks ago about avoiding an episiotomy but how do you know they remember? Bring extra copies of your birth plan to the birth to remind them about your wishes. Tell them again when you see them for the first time at the birth. They are human, you know.

12. **Some babies come out fast on their own, others ease out.** If the mother uses self-control. If possible, ease the baby out. Some women, especially first-time mothers, feel the baby come down into the vagina and overreact by screaming, "Get it out." They push with all their might forcing the baby to fly out and often tear in the process. Stay calm and let the baby do its thing.

The Creator is very efficient and it makes sense that He made the opening big enough as a general rule. With proper preparation prenatally, and good coaching while she pushes, most women do not need this procedure!

In May 2005 the *Journal of the American Medical Association* reported: "Evidence does not support maternal benefits traditionally ascribed to routine episiotomy. In fact, outcomes with episiotomy can be considered worse."

10

WHEN WILL THE BABY COME?

The question can be accurately answered in three words: "God only knows." As doctors we are far more concerned with how it comes than when it comes. As a husband you have, we realize, a special interest in the when.

This is like pointing to a particular little green apple developing on an apple tree and asking, "When will that particular apple ripen?" The appropriate answer is, "When it's ripe." Good farmers wait for the fruit to ripen. Good obstetricians do not "pick green apples." A good obstetrician has been defined as one equipped with a broad rear end and the good sense to sit calmly on it and let nature take its course.

PREMATURE BABIES

The rate of premature babies keeps increasing while the infant mortality rate does not seem to improve. In 2005 the United States had over half a million premature births. This is a 30 percent increase since 1981. On July 13, 2006, the National

Academy of Sciences, Institute of Medicine, estimated the cost of the care of premature babies at $26 billion a year. Many of these children will have continuing costly medical and educational challenges. Most of these children are medicated, and this cost would be a lot less if they were full-term, natural-childbirth babies.

Of course there are medical indications, in rare instances, that warrant interference and necessitate the forcing of labor before nature acts, such as maternal diabetes, severe Rh sensitization, etc., but these are indeed rare. We are not discussing these rare birds, but condemning any thought of forcing a normal baby to come for the convenience of the doctor, the parents, the impatient grandparents, or the thoughtlessly cruel neighbors who look at your wife's big abdomen and ask incredulously, "Haven't you had your baby yet?" then anxiously query, "What's wrong?" One experienced natural-childbirth mother got tired of friends and relatives phoning every day after she had gone beyond her due date, asking, "Are you still there?" She answered routinely, "No, this is a recording." Another was asked if she was still pregnant—she answered saucily, "Oh no! I'm carrying this baby around for a friend."

It can be especially nerve-racking to you and your wife if the pregnancy has extended beyond that calculated nine-month calendar date, called the "expected date of confinement," or due date. This ancient, ridiculously termed date is two weeks too early anyway—it is calculated upon the onset of your wife's last menstrual period, and even if she is one of those rare people who are accurate record keepers, she wasn't pregnant then anyway. Ovulation, and therefore conception, occurs about two weeks after menstruation. Because she can tell when she menstruates and can't tell when she ovulates (unless she's keeping a basal temperature record or studying cervical mucus or using one of the tests that predicts ovulation) down through the ages the calculation has been based upon the obvious sign. This sign, even with a record keeper, is not reliable.

REGULAR PERIODS

There's no such animal as a woman who always has regular periods. The ovulation doesn't always occur exactly two weeks after menstruation, as our Catholic friends who are depending upon the rhythm method know only too well. Sure as you count on it to, it won't.

GESTATION: 41½ WEEKS . . . NOT 40 WEEKS!

For years the expected date of confinement has been based on Naegele's rule. If you are interested in current literature you might be interested to know that Dr. Naegele died in the 1800s and we still use his rule. Some doctors are now giving due dates as thirty-seven weeks and calling this "at term." With over half a million premature babies being born each year, babies need to gestate completely until they are ready to be born. New research confirms our calculations. Average gestation is now known to be forty-one and one-seventh weeks, not forty weeks as previously thought (R. Mittendorf, et al., "The Length of Uncomplicated Human Gestation," *Obstetrics & Gynecology,* volume 75, number 6, June 1990).

To further confuse the calculation, some women may not miss their first, or even second, menstrual period when pregnant. We have had one mother who never missed a menstrual period throughout the entire length of pregnancy with three perfectly normal children.

CAN'T TELL BY FEELING

Any doctor who thinks he can feel your wife's abdomen and tell that the baby is "ready" is fooling himself. He will occasionally pull an apple that is still green, a baby that is not developed far enough to survive independently of its mother. The new ultra-sound method of determining fetal maturity has proven to be equally unreliable. God still only knows.

FALSE LABOR, YET IMPORTANT!

In the last months of pregnancy those aggravating false-labor cramps that make your wife uncomfortable do beneficial things to her baby and her cervix in preparation for the moment of birth. When a patient complains that she is having a lot of false labor, we smile peacefully and say, "Isn't that nice. Your uterus is getting your baby ready." The more false labor your wife has, the less real labor she will have, as these contractions are purposeful and beneficial. They soften and thin (efface) the cervix like kneading a piece of leather to make it more flexible so it will stretch better later. There are also hormones released by the placenta in the terminal stages of pregnancy that soften a hard cervix and prepare it for dilating.

The false labor contractions also benefit the passenger as well as the passageway. The intermittent squeezing and releasing of the baby makes the lungs more dilatable in preparation for taking over breathing when the time comes.

ONSET OF LABOR STILL IMPORTANT EVEN IF HAVING A CESAREAN

In the few women who have a contracted bony pelvis and must have a cesarean section, we still calmly sit and wait for the onset of labor, even though we know in advance that we are going to operate to get the baby. It would be more convenient for us, and the hospital personnel, if we scheduled the operation on a certain day, at a certain time. We refuse. God schedules a birthday, not man. The contractions of real labor tell us the baby is truly ready. They also help prevent hyaline membrane disease in the baby's lungs and respiratory distress syndrome (RDS) from incompletely developed lungs. Hyaline membrane disease occurs more often in babies delivered early or quickly (augmentation) or by cesarean section.

ADDITIONAL HELP

From the social and psychological standpoint we make two fervent pleas to you as a husband. First, get help with the housework (washing, cleaning, cooking, grocery shopping) for the first two weeks after a new baby is brought home. Let your wife give undivided tender loving care (TLC), as only a mother can, to the baby. Don't let her helper take care of the baby and your wife end up doing all the work. If the helper is your mother or her mother, she may be tempted to take over the baby—they are such cuddly little bundles of helplessness that her mother love will be aroused. Caring for a baby is best learned by doing, not by observing.

As the husband, sit down with your wife before the baby is born and make a list of things other people could do to help you. Bring food (that she likes), do a load or two of laundry, go shopping with a list, take toddlers to the park, clean, etc. Many women today want to do everything themselves and refuse help. Let's make it a tradition to help each other after having a baby. When someone calls and says, "Is there anything I can do?" the answer is, "Yes, I have a list." Your copy of *The Bradley Method Student Workbook* has helpful suggestions.

The second fervent plea we make is don't, please don't, call the helper to come until the baby is born. Why? There is nothing more productive of anxiety than someone hanging around uselessly, waiting for labor to start. They can undo in a few days all the self-confidence that months of training have accomplished. I recall one case of a nearly hysterical patient who related how her visiting mother paced the floor, wailing, "Oh, you poor dear, if I could just go through this for you." Don't condemn her. Remember, she didn't have natural childbirth. She may have had unmedicated, unattended childbirth, but she didn't have careful physical and psychological preparation during pregnancy from a Bradley class, and she didn't have a carefully trained husband-coach to guide her every step. No, don't condemn her; just don't invite her early and do send her a copy of this book to read in advance.

Even if she is a perfect angel and exudes calmness and confidence, she also has her own life to lead and you are wasting her time. You do not need her before the baby is born, you need her afterward. I can remember many distraught new mothers whose helper wouldn't take this advice and came, bag and baggage, on the calendar due date. But babies can't read calendars! The helper sat uselessly for two weeks, used up the vacation time she had allotted to help her daughter, then departed for home and employment just when the baby was born and she was needed.

Tell your helper what you know—the baby will come when it's good and ready and not until. Have her pass this information to her employer and get permission to start her two-week vacation when your wife calls and tells her she's had the baby.

OTHER CHILDREN IN THE FAMILY . . .
READ *CHILDREN AT BIRTH*

If you have other children, a practical suggestion is to make an agreement with a friend or neighbor to have them come over and take over your home as you leave for the hospital with your wife in labor. If this is the middle of the night, your friend or friends can simply go to sleep in your bed without disturbing the other children. Don't, as a husband and labor coach, try to dress and deliver the sleepy older children to someone else's house, because we need you. When the baby is born, call your helper, then go home and relieve your accommodating friend and wait for the helper to arrive.

Now, having planned a definite course of action for any conceivable day or time of day that your wife may go into real labor, let's explore the question again of when this will happen.

BELL-SHAPED CURVE

The length of pregnancy in any animal species if each case were plotted on a graph would result in a bell-shaped curve of normal incidence. For instance, let's plot a graph for, say, all the eight-pound babies born in your state for one year. (Of course, we mean the normal ones whose mothers are allowed to go to spontaneous labor.) The vertical arm of the graph would represent the number of babies, the horizontal arm the months of pregnancy. No matter where you lived on earth the curve would come out the same, bell-shaped. (See graph.)

This typical bell-shaped curve would result also if you similarly plotted the ripening of apples on a tree. A few would ripen early, a few late, and the majority would cluster around the central part of the curve. I thought of this same curve the other night while popping popcorn for the family. (My exasperated wife says I see natural-childbirth principles in everything!) All the popcorn kernels do not suddenly explode simultaneously with a single loud pop. Some start early, then more and more in a crescendo, then the number begins diminishing, with that last slowpoke kernel unexpectedly popping just as you go to pour the corn out, scattering kernels all over the kitchen.

Human babies follow the same pattern. Aggravating as it may be, that's the way it is, has been, and ever shall be with all of nature. There aren't very many eight-pound babies born at six months. The law of the perversity of nature usually takes over so that when one is, the mother got pregnant shortly after marriage, and how the neighbors' tongues wag. It would be as hard to convince them of this rare phenomenon as it was for me to convince a young sailor husband who got his wife pregnant on leave just before sailing overseas. The law of the perversity of nature manifested itself again, as this baby turned out to be one of those slow ones, far beyond the due date. Wouldn't you know!

I had to deal via the Red Cross with a distraught husband overseas, who bitterly claimed, "That couldn't be my kid," and a completely hysterical wife who was equally sure it couldn't be anyone else's. At which point along the curve will this particular baby of yours be placed? Again, only God knows.

MONTHS OF PREGNANCY

In healthy, normal mothers with healthy, normal babies there is no such thing as overdue. This term carries a dire connotation that unjustly scares the daylights out of uninformed people. More women have been unnecessarily forced into long, hard, unprepared labor, more babies damaged by being made to come through a tough, "green," unripe cervix, because everyone was ready except the baby. It takes an obstetrician with a firm backbone to withstand the onslaught from anxious relatives—"Why don't you do something? She's overdue!"

INDUCING LABOR

Before agreeing to have your baby induced think about the pros and cons and what drugs or procedures will be used. Go to www.fda.gov to check on drugs and their cautions or adverse effects. Ask your doctor what other choices you have and the pros and cons. Once you have the information, you know you made an informed decision.

I recall a couple whose long-standing problem of infertility was solved by the grace of God and basal temperature charts, cervical dilatation—in brief, the works. This most valuable baby turned out to be the slowest-growing one we have ever had. We were sure of the conception time via the basal temperature chart, or we would have assumed menstrual irregularities and a miscalculated due date. The mother went three months overdue and carried her baby a full year. We had no trouble with the grateful patient and her husband, but there were times during those three months when I thought my life was endangered— from the relatives and neighbors!

Sound obstetrical principles we will alter for no social reason. She finally went into spontaneous labor and had a six-and-a-half-pound baby. Why did it wait so long? I don't know.

BEYOND HER DUE DATE, DON'T WORRY ABOUT IT

If your wife goes beyond her due date, don't worry about it. You may want to try some of the tests for post-maturity, like the biophysical profile, etc., or talk to your pediatrician. They may reassure you and reduce your stress. But remember, these tests are not 100 percent accurate. The tests themselves may have a negative effect on your baby. Do take your wife out more often to be with friends. Get her mind off herself and her baby by distracting her with interesting things to do, interesting people to meet, interesting places to go. Remind her, gently, that the baby will come when it is ready.

HOW TO RECOGNIZE REAL LABOR

This sometimes takes a bit of doing, especially if your wife has had previous children. First, let's reassure both of you: it is rare to have a woman in real labor who doesn't know she's in real labor. Early labor can be difficult to recognize but real (active) labor is pretty hard to ignore. Assuming you are going to a hospital or birth center that supports and respects the principles of natural childbirth, once you know it's real labor, get there. Some doctors want to be called first before you leave, others don't. Find out this little detail during your pregnancy. My associates and I are the variety who plead, "If you know it's real labor—don't call, get to the hospital."

The reason we don't want our patients to phone if they know they are in real labor is for their own benefit. If the phone call comes in during the night, our telephone secretary may have to reply, "The doctor is tied up in the delivery room now. I'll have him call you when he's free." So the couple sits at home, labor getting harder and harder, waiting for the return call. As they sit and wait I've often wondered just what they expect the doctor to say when he calls. I've often been tempted when a patient says on the phone, "I'm in hard labor, what'll I do?" to answer, "Well, you could take in a movie, you could visit friends, you could go shopping, but then perhaps it would be a better idea to come to the hospital if you know you're going to have a baby!" We do not yield to temptation but simply say, "Come to the hospital."

If they had minded our rule in the first place, this delay would not have occurred. While we were finishing up the other case she could have been prepped by the nurse before the labor became so advanced. Remember, relaxation promotes rapid progressive dilatation of the cervix.

I recall one exasperated husband who made a great contribution to our efficiency by asking us why in Hades we hadn't given his wife that long, complicated hospital admission form for him to fill out during her many office visits? They could have filled it out leisurely at home and had her bring it back. Good idea! That's what we now do. He was exasperated because he missed the birth and very much wanted to be there. He was downstairs filling out the form when she gave birth shortly after arriving. As it turned out, it was their own fault this occurred. She had had three previous babies after long, hard labors, and frankly they didn't believe the principles of natural childbirth one bit. They had decided to try it only because "nothing could be worse" than what she had experienced before.

When labor had started at home they decided to experiment with it at home to see if it made any difference to relax, breathe with the abdomen, etc. May I make the plea again, don't do this, for two reasons. One, if you wish to experiment, that's perfectly all right, but do it in the hospital, it's more efficient. Two, you're taking unnecessary chances of not making it to the hospital. This couple "tried out" the principles at home and barely made it.

Start for the hospital as soon as your wife is convinced that she is in actual labor for another reason—so you can drive carefully and not have to hurry. Under no, repeat, no conditions should you exceed the speed limit, run through red lights, or otherwise take silly chances driving. Some frantic, untrained husband ran through a red light in our city and killed two occupants of another car, and his wife had the baby the next day. Police rightly take a dim view of disobeying traffic laws because your wife is in labor. Should the rare occurrence happen that your wife has the baby in the car—let her, and you keep driving calmly to the hospital. What do you do with the baby? Nothing. Errors committed are always errors of commission, not errors of omission. Your wife can pick it up and put it to her breast and cuddle it if she wishes, should the trip be rather long, but you do not need to cut or tie the cord, or try to deliver the placenta, or do anything else except be a chauffeur.

These babies and mothers do beautifully, remember. Doctors are necessary when babies won't come, not when they so readily do. All husbands think this might happen to them, but let me reassure you it rarely does. It has happened only three times in my medical career and wouldn't have then if the parents had obeyed the simple rules. It is annoying how often the late ones are parents who live only a few blocks away from the hospital, yet the ones who live at a great distance get there in time.

I recall one hilarious scene at the emergency-room entrance as the nurse and I attended such an occurrence. The experienced natural-childbirth mother was sitting, tailor fashion, in the backseat of the car in her gown. She was holding the baby to her breast, the umbilical cord intact, the placenta still in place. Her eyes were bright with merriment as she looked at the baby and exclaimed, "Look, isn't he cute?" Then she broke into peals of laughter at her husband's discomfiture. We knew they lived nearby and found out that labor had started two hours before. Why hadn't they started sooner? The mother answered brightly, "I was watching a murder mystery on TV and I waited to see 'who dun it'!"

There are certain handicaps in teaching the self-confidence of natural childbirth to mothers. One of our teachers, Rhondda Hartman, strolled in calmly with her third baby just ready to be born. Why hadn't she come sooner? we asked. The nonchalant answer was, "I was busy. The La Leche League meeting was at my house tonight." She had calmly finished her job as hostess first, and then, oh, yes, dropped by to have the baby. Her other children think babies are born at home. She had tucked them in, had the other babies during the night, and gone back home two hours after each birth to greet them in the morning with the new baby. She, like the other teachers, practices what she preaches. There is no problem, then, if your wife knows she is in labor. Simply come to the hospital.

IF YOU'RE NOT SURE . . .

Now, what if your wife doesn't know, just suspects or thinks maybe? Try going through this list of activities:

1. Have a snack.
2. Have something to drink (water, juice, etc.).
3. Go for a walk.
4. Take a warm shower or bath (as long as the bag of waters is intact).
5. Take a nap. Feel free to call your doctor or midwife and discuss it with them. Obstetricians don't mind being called at odd hours or they wouldn't be obstetricians. The rewards are magnificent, but the hours are terrible!

EACH BIRTH IS DIFFERENT

Some labors begin with far-apart contractions, some with close-together ones. The only thing we are sure of, as doctors, is that they are all different. No two labors are exactly alike, even with the same mother. This has been objectively demonstrated by recordings from a tocodynamometer (like the uterine-monitor part of an external fetal monitor), a gadget that makes graphs of the uterine muscle activity. In thousands of graphs no two were exactly alike. If your wife has had previous babies, don't judge by what happened last time and expect it to be the same this time. It isn't necessarily so. It may be very different this time.

If her uterine contractions are coming ten minutes apart or less in their regularity, then do they meet the next requirement: Are they progressively harder? Are they picking up and getting stronger? Ask her. Some episodes of false labor have mild contractions that may be less than ten minutes apart. If you apply the tests below, these false contractions will usually fade out and quit. But if her contractions meet these requirements, get her to the hospital without further delay. Other signs you as the husband can look at are the emotional signposts, length of contractions, mother's modesty as listed in *The Bradley Method Student Workbook*.

If there is doubt in your mind or hers, then you have time to apply the following tests. If the questionable labor began while your wife was up and around, she should do the pelvic rock (horizontal variety) exercise for a while and then lie down in the side position, curled up in a ball, as previously described. If the questionable labor began during the night while she was reclining or sleeping, she should get up and walk about for a while. In other words, she should change her activity to the opposite of what she was doing.

If it was only false labor, the effect of this change will be to make the contractions less strong, further apart, and more irregular. Get out your watch and time them (from the start of one to the start of another) before and after the change. If they are further apart and she feels that they are not as strong, wait awhile and see what happens. They may increase later or they may completely fizzle out. If this change of activity does not affect them and they continue to get more regular, closer, and progressively harder, come to the hospital. Sometimes that old law of the perversity of nature catches up with us.

Your wife may meet the test fully at home, and yet the uterine activity may stop after she gets to the hospital. This may be a result of the effects of adrenaline on labor. Adrenaline can be caused by anxiety, excitement, fear, etc. For reasons that aren't too clear to me, this seems to upset the parents. They act embarrassed and apologize profusely to the doctor or nurse for having bothered them. Let me assure you false labor doesn't bother the baby, the doctor, or the nurses. Don't let it bother you if it should happen.

Please take notice I haven't mentioned two phenomena as being part of the indication of true labor. Some patients have the preconceived notion that the water has to break before true labor begins. This is most assuredly not so; some babies are "born with the veil" as it was called in olden times. The water may never break. The baby is pushed out still contained in its intact bag of waters. (I believe superstition has it that babies so born are destined to be great leaders.) Usually the water bag doesn't break until late in labor.

BAG OF WATERS BREAKS

But if it does break at home, and believe me you'll know this if it happens, call your doctor or midwife or go to the hospital, or if it's during regular hours some doctors prefer that you stop at the office. If the water has appeared in a large amount it doesn't matter whether your wife is having uterine contractions or not or what nature they may be—come anyway.

If this happens, be ready to tell your doctor or midwife what is happening. The water broke. What does it look like? A spot on the sheets, or is it running down her leg? Color? It should be clear and may have some white specks or a little blood in it. If it is brown, or green, or any color, it is a problem. What does it smell like? It should smell like nothing or salt water. If it smells funny or putrid, it is a problem. What is the baby doing? Is it moving normally? That is what it should be doing. How does the mother feel? Perhaps a little excited, that would be normal but does she feel sick or like she has the flu? What would indicate a problem?

Then remind your doctor or midwife what they said at your last visit. Did they say the baby had dropped or engaged? If the baby has already engaged they might feel better. Then reassure them you are calm and the mother would like to take a shower and a nap and you will call them later. This is why you have a team so you can discuss these things and know that you can trust them to help you make a wise decision.

KNOWING WHY HELPS YOU REMEMBER TO DO

Why? You're more likely to remember to do something if you know why, our principles of natural childbirth dictate. Here's why:

1. The umbilical cord may come down and out with the water. If this happens, the presenting part of the baby may put pressure on the cord and compromise the baby's lifeline. The mother may be asked to get on all fours with her head down. The doctor or nurse wants to listen to your baby's heartbeat (this gives a clue) or if needed check the cervix to tell by feeling if the cord came down (there is additional danger of infection with a vaginal exam). He or she will know what to do if this rare thing occurs.

2. She's liable to start hard labor shortly. Not every woman has labor shortly after the water breaks, but most do. It is noted for being hard, fast, and effective on most occasions. Or putting it another way, you'll probably have to go to the hospital shortly anyway, so you might as well start right away. Get a bath towel to catch the flow of salt water. Sanitary napkins are too small. The salt water comes in intermittent gushes, and some gushes can be quite profuse.

   Some mothers are suspicious that their water may have broken but are not sure. This confusion arises from liquefied mucous plugs of the cervix suddenly letting go, and by a tendency in late pregnancy, after the baby has "dropped," to have slight involuntary leakage of urine. These slow leaks are a nuisance and may be a small high leak in the bag of waters or urine, but do not yield anywhere near the quantity of fluid present when the water bag really gives way.

This very seldom happens prior to labor, let me repeat. We are amazed that it doesn't happen more often, when you consider how thin and fragile-looking the amniotic sac is and how powerful the uterine muscle is.

APPEARANCE OF BLOOD

The second phenomenon that does not have to happen to be true labor is the appearance of blood in the vaginal secretions. We have had patients get this preconceived notion from their grandmother, or some equally unreliable source, and sit at home trying to ignore progressively harder uterine contractions because they couldn't believe it was real labor as they hadn't had a "bloody show," as it is called. Bleeding isn't necessary. Its absence does not mean it's not labor, nor does its presence necessarily mean it is labor. All this little dab of bleeding means to a doctor is that the woman is pregnant, and probably has been pregnant before.

Heavy bleeding, as much as a menstrual flow, is a definite abnormality and should be reported to your doctor at once.

The little bloody "spotting" we are discussing comes from the stretching or thinning of the cervix from the effect of pre-labor. There is much more likelihood of little spots of blood accompanying this if the cervix has previously been stretched with a baby's passage. It can happen occasionally even with the first baby. It usually happens in the last month especially in multiparas (women who have had previous babies), but can happen anytime in the last three months. It is caused by the false labor, or Braxton-Hicks, contractions working on the cervix to prepare it for dilatation. It does not necessarily mean that the baby is coming early or soon. It is a most unreliable sign of anything, except pregnancy in the last three months.

BACKACHE OR LOWER ABDOMINAL CRAMPS . . . UNRELIABLE SIGN

Backache or lower abdominal cramps are also an unreliable sign of labor. Some labors, depending on the position and size of the baby, have very little backache involved—it's all in front. And vice versa, again depending on the position and size of the baby, the ache may be all in the back, and very little in the front. Pay attention to the original requirements of uterine contractions. Feel the uterus, see what it is doing, (it should be moving forward during contractions), time it, ask your wife if it is progressively contracting harder—these indications are not always reliable, either.

A TRIP THROUGH THE HOSPITAL—IN ADVANCE

This isn't necessary, it is just nice. There is a Birth Place Tour form in *The Bradley Method Student Workbook,* which will give you questions to ask. If your hospital has a conducted tour to acquaint you with the facilities, avail yourself of it, both you and your wife.

FAMILIARIZE YOURSELF

Become familiar with which door you enter, especially after daylight hours. Get an admission form beforehand and have it all filled out in advance. Take the tour through the delivery-room section. Have the unfamiliar-looking paraphernalia shown and explained to you in advance. Take the tour through the labor-room section. Become familiar with the place so that when you arrive with your wife in labor you won't wander aimlessly around, wondering where to go.

BIRTHING ROOMS AND LDR ROOMS

Ask about birthing rooms and LDR rooms. What are the criteria for inclusion or exclusion—do you have to be a certain number of centimeters dilated? Bag of waters broken? Meconium in water? Ask lots of questions so you know what you are facing.

PRIOR ARRANGEMENTS

Probably the most important thing you can do to help your wife stay calm and peaceful as she enters labor is to make prior arrangements for the financial coverage of her stay. Hospital admissions offices will have very little sympathy for husbands who had nine long months to make financial arrangements for their wives, then pull that stupid "emergency" idea when their wives go into labor. I've seen perfectly prepared mothers break down in embarrassment and all their preparation go to naught because their husbands had to argue with the admissions office to get them in.

INSURANCE

If you have insurance, bring your policy, visit the admissions office as early as possible during your wife's pregnancy, and make all arrangements. I can't think of a better way to honor the woman you love than to give her the secure feeling you are taking care of her in every way.

NATURAL CHILDBIRTH IS LESS EXPENSIVE

There are multiple advantages of unmedicated natural childbirth. One of these, you will discover to your pleasure, is less hospital expense. There is no anesthetist's fee when there is no anesthetist. Also, the comparatively short stay of unmedicated mothers and babies can reduce the bill. Neither mother nor baby is sick, and their stay can be shortened. Think of how much money we could save in our health-care system if more mothers chose natural childbirth. Remember to bring *The Bradley Method Student Workbook* and the birth plan you worked on in class.

11

POSTPARTUM AND FAMILY RELATIONS

After having the baby and drinking the iced orange juice, the original birthday party refreshment given as a reward to natural-childbirth parents, parents usually inquire: "When can we go home?"

HOSPITAL STAY

How long should your wife stay in the hospital? The answer to that is as long as she wishes. How long should the baby stay in the hospital? The answer here is, barring prematurity or complications, as short a time as possible. Why? As Dr. Thaddeus Montgomery has stated, "The hospital is a good place to deliver a baby but a poor place to board it" (T. L. Montgomery, *American Journal of Obstetrics & Gynecology,* volume 81, 1961, pp. 890–901).

ROOMING-IN FACILITIES

Most hospitals today have rooming-in facilities, the only hurry to get the baby out would be financial. The rent comes high. If they don't have rooming-in facilities, then get the baby home as soon as possible. What's the hurry? Because of the mixing of bacteria from other babies by putting them all in a large nursery together. I care not how "sterile" the technique, this is bacteriologically ridiculous. Babies don't get infections from themselves or their mothers (they are born with acquired immunity to most mother's bacteria); they get them from other babies. Also, babies cannot read hospital feeding schedules. They want to eat on their own schedule and this very rarely happens to coincide with the nursery's schedule—as evidenced by their frustrated crying.

EIGHTEEN-MONTH GESTATIONS . . . NINE IN AND NINE OUT

Ashley Montagu has a theory that the human infant really has a gestational period of eighteen months, and that the only reason the human being is born after nine months of gestation is because of the size of its head and brain in comparison to other animals. If you look at other animals' development, you'll note the human does not catch up with other animals until around nine months of age. Because of this he suggests that perhaps the human really is an extragestational fetus. This means the baby needs as much love, care, and attention the first nine months outside the uterus as it did the first nine months inside the uterus. Perhaps we should think of ourselves as marsupials.

DO NOT SEPARATE

For psychological reasons babies should stay with their mothers. The best person to care for the baby is its mother. The nurses may be the best nurses available, but they are not the mother. And don't think that baby of yours doesn't notice the difference.

Moms, babies, and dads have a stronger bond if they are close right after birth, than if they are separated. This bonding is critical in order to increase the love relationship and avoid rejection, as occurs in other animals separated from their young.

Later on, your baby may have to be temporarily separated from his mother. But the first two weeks of life, especially the first few hours and days, represent an extreme change in his life to which he must adjust.

Imagine for a while the nature of the changes in his world that occurred at birth. From 98.6-degree warmth to 70-degree room temperature. From total darkness to glaring overhead lights in the hospital. From relative quiet, where instead of Mother's familiar voice and the soothing rhythmical sounds of her body (her heartbeat, breath sounds, etc.) there are sudden loud, unfamiliar, startling noises. From being carried constantly with the rocking motion from Mother's hip movements, to the utter stillness of a crib. From soft, smooth, saltwater feelings to dry, sterile, harsh sheets (you may see a red rash on the baby's skin from contact). From being fed continuously from Mother's body via the lifeline, or cord, to being on a schedule. Can you blame any baby for wanting to go home with Mother? For wanting to be loved, and held, and rocked, and talked to, and fed when hungry?

Now, what about the mother? We find the mother who gets to hold and breast-feed her baby immediately after it is born, and who does not have her baby taken from her to be put in what I sarcastically call the "kid concentration camp," or hospital nursery, has not only a more psychologically stable baby, but is herself a far better, more loving mother.

The benefits of togetherness of mother and baby are reciprocal. There are many, many benefits of giving birth without medication of any nature, but the greatest benefit of all is probably that an unmedicated natural-childbirth mother can be trusted to have her baby with her and to care for it immediately when it is born, whereas a mother who has had any medication—I care not how supposedly small the dose—is mentally confused, recovering from an epidural, or "drunk" from drugs, and may not be trusted with the baby.

If complications occurred, justifying the giving of drugs, then this is purposeful and necessary. With proper training of husband and wife, most of the mothers neither need nor ask for drugs and the exuberant, alert, capable mother is perfectly able to handle, hold, and care for her baby. She needs no substitute mother and eagerly accepts her baby.

SEPARATION DECREASES MOTHERLINESS

Although we cannot make a direct comparison with lower animals, only indirect, anyone working with animals is familiar with the fact that if the babies are separated from the mothers at birth, the length of separation results in decreasing degrees of motherliness upon return of the infant, and if separation is too long, the mother will totally reject the infant. Dr. Marshall Klaus published a study on whether human mothers have this "sensitive period" (bonding) immediately after delivery as has been reported among animal mothers (Klaus et al., "Maternal Attachment," *New England Journal of Medicine*, volume 286, March 2, 1972, pp. 440–463).

REJECTION OF OFFSPRING

In goats, cows, and sheep, separation of the mother and her offspring immediately after birth for a period of as short as one or two hours often resulted in unmother-like behavior and rejection of the offspring. She may butt him away or feed him and other infants indiscriminately. Dr. Klaus said that, in contrast, if the animal mother and offspring are together for the first few days of this sensitive period and are then separated for several days and reunited, the mother quickly resumes her protective role.

Dr. Klaus found that human mothers who were allowed

contact with their babies in this sensitive period were more responsive to their infants' needs, were reluctant to leave them in the care of others, and showed greater sensitivity to the infants' cries and made greater efforts to soothe them. It seems then that we can make comparisons between human mothers and the other animals in ways other than the conduct of labor.

HOME BEST FOR RESTING

The mother needs rest after laboring, but have you ever been around a hospital long? She will rest far better in her own familiar bed at home, hearing the familiar noises she is so accustomed to, as opposed to clanging bedpans, squawking call systems, talking personnel, patients, and visitors. For goodness' sake, go home. Remember to have a helper there to do the work; with this arrangement most mothers would rather be home.

NATURAL-CHILDBIRTH MOMS CAN GO HOME TWO HOURS AFTER BIRTH

Unmedicated mothers and unmedicated normal-size babies are not sick and do far better at home. The average stay for natural-childbirth patients in our hospital is less than twenty-four hours. A few of our athletes insist on going immediately after the two-hour period of observation following the birth. In the absence of medication or complication we have always allowed this—if they are breast-feeding and they have help at home. We know the nursing will keep the postpartum uterus tight.

ADJUSTMENT PERIOD

After arriving home there will be a period of adjustment for the husband. The "little stranger," as Grandmother called the baby, can surely disrupt the interpersonal relationship between you and your wife—as you remembered it. She hardly ever has time for you. She will later, so don't let it throw you. Now look at the place! If there are housekeeping chores to do, do more than your share. Hold your horses; cooperation is the key. There just isn't time enough when the baby is so little. Don't be demanding and expect your former harmony to be restored immediately. Plan on being the cook if you aren't already, or resort to takeout—baby takes precedence. Later on things will get back to schedule, so cheer up!

SEX

Lovemaking? She can't be bothered with it now, psychologically or physically. Wait—for about four weeks. After her postpartum check at four weeks the doctor will plan with her the method of choice for spacing her pregnancies if she so desires. Babies are bundles of joy, but not when they come every nine months!

LUBRICATION

There may be occasions when there is reduced vaginal mucus because of hormone fluctuation from birth and breast-feeding. This may affect comfortable intercourse during the course of breast-feeding. This is somewhat similar to extra dryness just after menstrual flow. Have on hand a tube of K-Y jelly to aid as a lubricant. It is the same water-soluble lubricant we doctors use for gloves and vaginal instruments and can be purchased from the druggist without a prescription.

NOT IGNORED . . . ADDITIONAL FAMILY OBLIGATIONS

Well, what can you do? In the midst of all this female activity you may feel a little lost and left out, and definitely ignored on occasions. Rest assured that just your presence makes a great difference. She knows you're around. She appreciates your presence, help, and love, even if she doesn't always say so.

What happened to your role as a coach? It's still there. Let's review some of the things you can coach and remind your wife to do now, as you did during pregnancy and labor.

PHYSICAL FACTORS

Your wife's three B muscles (Back, Belly, Bottom) have done their duty, but they have been necessarily stretched and weakened from use. They need to be strengthened and tightened to restore her to the nonpregnant shape. The postpartum exercises are nearly identical to the prepartum, with the addition of more vigorous abdominal exercises. There was no point during pregnancy of trying to draw in abdominal muscles that were steadily stretching out.

COLD OR ICE PACKS

For comfort most doctors recommend wrapped cold or ice packs on and off the perineum the first day and sitz baths after that. Again, the ancient idea that your wife can't take a bath has been shown to be ridiculous. She should take a long, warm, leisurely bath twice a day for two weeks, then once daily. The penetrating heat of soaking a part of your body is more beneficial and effective than surface heat. If she had stitches, this will help healing.

MENSTRUAL FLOW

The lochial drainage (vaginal menstrual flow) is normal for about a month following the birth. Right after birth and if she goes out in public for long periods, she should wear two pads for protection because the discharge may come in irregular amounts and it's hard to tell when the extra pad is necessary. At home after the first few days a single pad is all that is needed. Avoid tampons or sea sponges at this time.

EXTERNAL VAGINAL SKIN

The external vaginal skin needs protection from moisture and infection. Bathing this area should be done without soap, just as before the baby. Once everything has healed, most doctors further suggest that she use the same lotion preparation on herself that she uses on her baby. The same application is suggested for the same reason, to prevent diaper rash in the baby and to prevent panty rash in the mother. If she really wants healthy skin in this area, she should abstain from panties for life.

VITAMINS AND SUPPLEMENTS

She should continue the same vitamin and iron supplementary pills that were prescribed during pregnancy, at least until the doctor checks her at four weeks and as long as she continues to breast-feed.

EXERCISES

These are essentially a repetition of the prenatal ones, like tailor sitting and Kegeling when she can. Encourage her to use common sense and begin doing these exercises when she feels comfortable doing them. Now, with a new baby, she will have additional opportunities to utilize these beneficial exercises. Baby's diapers may be changed on the floor. She should put an extra baby blanket on the floor and tailor sit with the baby while Kegeling.

Your wife won't need to do any extra tailor sitting; just taking care of the baby will give her plenty of opportunity.

Sitting on a hard floor, even if carpeted, sounds uncomfortable if your wife has had stitches, but it only sounds that way. Actually, she will be more uncomfortable sitting on a soft seat. Why? Because on the firm floor she sits down on her sitting-down bones of her pelvis (ischial tuberosities), and these aren't sore, as the stitches aren't near them. The stitches are in the flesh up between these bony prominences, and the floor doesn't hit the sensitive area as a cushion or soft seat would.

PELVIC ROCKING

The pelvic rocking should be done before getting in bed at night—for the rest of her life. Professional models, movie stars, and others do this to keep their bodies and posture beautiful. Your wife's body is just as important. If "after pains" become a nuisance at home, she should pelvic rock and curl up on her side at intervals during the day. She will not only look better, she will feel better.

"RUNNING" POSITION

The "running" position of sleep—on her side with top leg pulled up—is equally applicable for the rest of her life after having the baby! In the immediate postpartum period it seems to allow the still-heavy uterus to fall freely forward, which is important in preventing a backward or "tipped" uterus from developing.

KEGEL

The exercise for the Kegel (vaginal, bladder, and rectal) muscle should be continued as during the pregnancy. A good additional time to perform it is while she is nursing or feeding the baby. Ask her if she's doing it and remind her to do it regularly.

The abdominal muscles need the most attention, as they were stretched the most over the longest period of time. The time for performing extra or deliberate abdominal muscle exercises is on awakening. It took nine months to stretch those muscles, remember, and it takes nine months to tighten them. Accordingly, set your alarm clock ten minutes earlier for the next nine months after the baby comes and you and your wife do these deliberate abdominal muscle calisthenics every morning during this period. Do them with her, you ask? It won't hurt you to have a flatter stomach, too!

After two weeks of continuous TLC (tender loving care) of the baby, take your wife out once a week for the rest of your life together. Get a babysitter or take the baby with you. When she feels ready try a sport that involves great vigor. Swimming is ideal. Golf, tennis, square dancing, bowling, walking—it doesn't matter which. What did you do before the baby? Do it again, and do it regularly. Social exercises, participating with a group of friends, are not only more fun but more likely to be regularly pursued. Calisthenics at home get boring.

ACTIVITY

How much activity should your wife have after having a baby? Whatever she feels like. Just as during pregnancy, she will tire more rapidly. Having a baby is hard work and she has donated a portion of her reserve energy to her baby—that's where the baby got it. Her reserves will gradually build up. They will build up more rapidly if she returns to her usual type of conduct. Again, she may not immediately be able to swim as many laps or bowl as many games as before her pregnancy. This does not mean she shouldn't indulge and should become a sedentary figure. It means she should stop and rest when she tires. She'll decide.

UP AND DOWN STEPS

There is a silly superstition that she shouldn't go up and down steps after having a baby. She shouldn't have to go up and down steps constantly. It would be helpful if the house could be re-arranged somewhat so that items she needs frequently are kept on the same level. But she can go up and down steps if she takes her time about it and doesn't overtire herself.

DRIVING

Another silly superstition is that women can't drive cars after having babies. If she is an experienced driver, there is no earthly reason why not. In fact, she should have a car available for her own use, now that she has a baby. Household supplies may run out and she may need to shop more often to meet the baby's needs. Also, she shouldn't feel tied down so she can't go any-where. She will tend to blame this tied-down feeling on the baby, when it's just lack of transportation. And babies love to ride in their car seats. Check with your local stores or places like www.safeandsecurebaby.com for current information on laws, proper use, and installation of car seats. The older and more rick-ety the car, the more it vibrates and rattles, the more babies like it. If you want to soothe a colicky, fussy baby, take it for a ride in the car. The rhythmical vibrations of the motor tend to soothe it.

SUGGESTED BOOKS

All parents have misgivings about their parenting capabilities. These are magnified by reading the confusing multitude of books advising parents. Limit this reading to avoid confusion.

I would suggest these books as being perfectly adequate for ready reference on any problems that may arise:

The Baby Book, by William Sears, M.D., and Martha Sears, R.N. with Robert and James Sears (Little, Brown and Co., 2003)

How to Raise a Healthy Child In Spite of Your Doctor, by Robert Mendelsohn, M.D. (Ballentine Books, 1987)

The Womanly Art of Breastfeeding, by La Leche League
   (Plume, 2004)
Good Nights: The Happy Parents' Guide to the Family Bed,
   by Jay Gordon, M.D. (St. Martin's Griffin, 2002)
*Sweet Dreams: A Pediatrician's Secrets for Baby's Good
   Nights' Sleep,* by Paul Fleiss, M.D. (McGraw-Hill, 2000).

Some of these books may be out of print, but available at your
library. Consult your doctor, midwife, or pediatrician about
anything that can't be cleared up by the advice in these books.

FIRST BABY?

If this is your first baby, remember the old saying: babies grow
up in spite of the parents, not due to them. Your only real responsibility is to "have 'em, love 'em, and leave 'em be." Let
them be little individuals. Don't try to force your preconceived
notions of what you think they ought to do or be upon them as
they grow. Let them be themselves, and take joy in the privilege
of being with them for a while. In the steadily increasing life
span of both of you the period during which children are dependent upon you is, proportionately, very short. Enjoy it. They
begin to acquire independence surprisingly early. They need
guidance and chaperoning, of course, but don't try to make a
round peg fit in a square hole. Let them be what they are, not
what you think they ought to be.

Children who have their needs met as infants tend to grow up
to be independent children and adults. Clinging children often
are ones who did not have their needs met when they were
young and may grow up to be clinging adults.

Parents who foster feelings of indebtedness and overdepen-
dency in their children are reflecting their own sense of inade-
quacy. Be someone in your own right and let your children do
likewise. They will admire and respect you in adulthood as they
loved you in childhood.

It goes without saying that babies need their mothers' full-time love, nourishment, and attention especially during the first few years of life. No one can adequately substitute for her. Be creative and try to find ways to be with your baby during this special formative time. Many couples tell me they had to reevaluate their priorities and reduce expenses, choose less expensive extras or eliminate them. Home-based opportunities may be the answer. If you have to return to work—take as much time off as you can. Continue breast-feeding and read about working and parenting in *The Baby Book,* by Dr. Sears.

EDUCATION

Encourage her to continue her education via the many wonderful opportunities for adult education. You might study some together. Maintain other interests in order to avoid a psychological feeling of having outlived her usefulness that can make menopause a period of great depression. The key is to keep those interests up when her children are little and have fun with them at all ages. I know some women who take college classes with their kids. You might enjoy becoming a Bradley teacher, and changing the lives of other families.

Housework, children, and life can be very rewarding, but no one should lose their individuality. Families are a lot of work and a lot of fun.

12

HUSBAND'S ROLE IN BREAST-FEEDING

We have taken note of the famous slogan that contented cows give better milk. Nervousness interferes with milk formation in human mothers, too. We have finally found the main cause of nervousness in women—men.

As specialists in teaching women natural childbirth, we have found the cooperation of husbands indispensable. Statistics illustrate the importance of togetherness at this time. The BEST labor companion is the husband when Bradley trained. Obstetricians who tried to forbid the participation of husbands and hospitals that excluded them from the delivery room had more anxious, frightened mothers who pleaded for medication and required more forceps deliveries, and cesareans.

The same holds for breast-feeding. The success of breast-feeding will be affected by the attitude of the husband toward it. His attitude will depend, in turn, upon experiences in his past, even early childhood, in relationship to breast-feeding.

I recall one young couple on their first visit in the office, in the wife's first pregnancy. I asked the wife if she planned to breast-feed her baby. She never had a chance to answer. The husband shot out of his chair and declared in a hostile tone, "She is not." I looked surprised and asked why not. "I married her because of her breasts, they're mine, and I'm not going to have any kid touching them, including my own!" He was only expressing openly what a lot of men unknowingly manage to convey in subtle ways to subconsciously discourage their wives.

Could such exaggerated importance of the breasts be related to his frustration from early weaning, or bottle-feeding, or perhaps the power of suggestion from every book cover, billboard, and auto-tire advertisement? What a basis for marriage!

WHY ENCOURAGE YOUR WIFE TO BREAST-FEED?

Let's start from scratch. Why should you subtly or openly encourage your wife to nurse her baby? What difference does it make? To whom? Is there some magic in mother's milk? As men, we must admit that breasts do make lovely sweater decorations. However, as doctors, we remind you that their primary purpose is a source of food, and immunities for babies. Any part of the human body is healthier when used properly for its intended purpose. Cancer of the breast occurs less in breasts that have been used to feed babies. A January 30, 2001, report from the Associated Press reported, "Women who breast fed their babies for two years or longer reduced their risk of breast cancer by 50 percent. . . ."

As a doctor, an obstetrician, the benefits I seek are primarily to your wife. However, there are selfish reasons why we natural-childbirth-oriented obstetricians prefer your wife to breast-feed her baby, particularly in the "sensitive period" (bonding) immediately after birth. In the olden days, when a mother was drugged or paralyzed, the doctor could push on the mother's abdomen and bear down on the uterus, squeezing and pushing to make the placenta leave the uterus.

BREAST-FEEDING SEPARATES THE PLACENTA

With unmedicated mothers, this would be most uncomfortable, so we are dependent on the mother to separate the placenta naturally by breast-feeding the baby. Fewer placentas are trapped this way, as the stimulation of breast-feeding causes expulsive waves of natural uterine contractions that begin at the top of the uterus and progressively work downward, serving to expel the placenta. Oxytocic drugs tend to cause tetanic contractions of the uterus as a whole, occurring at once, that trap and retain the placenta.

TWINS

Breast-feeding can make a big difference with twins. Our statistics on the management of multiple pregnancies, twins, and so forth, are most beautiful because, first, we have such big babies, thanks to good nutrition and the natural-childbirth exercises.

Second, our mothers don't even associate having babies with being drugged.

Third, we again imitate nature in management of labor—after all, most other mammals have more than one infant at a time—in that we put each baby to breast when it is born, allowing the mother to handle it, skin to skin, immediately. This serves the normal purpose of stimulating the uterus to produce expulsive waves of contractions from above downward to produce the next infant.

At a professionals' seminar held under the auspices of our American Academy of Husband-Coached Childbirth, one of our leotard-clad teacher models was a lovely artist, Panchita MacNeil, at term pregnancy with known twins and her slim, lovely body performed the prenatal exercises for the assembled group very nicely in spite of a very distended abdomen. A few days later, under the coaching of her husband, Ron, with encouragement from her natural-childbirth-oriented obstetrician,

Arnold Bresky, M.D., she calmly gave birth naturally to the first baby who was breech (six pounds, fourteen ounces) and put it to her breast, which stimulated the uterus to push the next baby (seven pounds, two ounces) into the vertex, or headfirst, position.

She then happily gave birth naturally to the second one, put it to her breast, thereby causing spontaneous passage of the two placentas, and from the efficient uterine contractions stimulated by the breast-feeding, the uterus tightened down, shutting off the maternal sinuses at the placental site—all this with hardly a drop of blood being wasted by the uterus. She then had her orange juice and walked out of the birth room. Mother Nature is efficient when utilized. Our directors, Jay and Marjie Hathaway, took movies of the births to illustrate natural-childbirth management of twins, utilizing breast-feeding by the undrugged, cooperative mother as a stimulus to the uterus.

BENEFITS

What are other benefits of breast-feeding? Let's consider a few. We think the Creator intended that your wife should not have an immediate return of her menstrual bleeding after having a baby. She has donated blood to the baby itself (not directly but via the ingredients), the blood does not cross the placenta but O_2, nutrients, and many essential items do and she then loses some incident to birth. The recovery phase from this loss after the baby is born should not be handicapped by menstruation. It's hard to build up a depleted savings account when regular withdrawals are made. The breasts' hormones serve to delay menstruation by suppressing ovulation after the baby is born. Some women may have menstrual periods while breast-feeding (even these are lighter!), but most women do not.

Men hardly ever have low levels of iron and oxygen (hemoglobin) in their blood, but many women do. Breast-feeding mothers have higher blood iron levels than mothers who bottle-feed. They are generally more energetic, feel better, and are more fun to live with and be around.

SHRINKING OF UTERUS

The uterus contracts by reflex during breast-feeding. This causes it to shrink back (involute) faster to its nonpregnant size. This means less backache, pelvic dragging feeling, varicose veins, etc., from a big, heavy uterus.

CALMING EFFECT, MORE MOTHERLY

Then there is the psychological effect of this "womanly art" on your wife. When the milk comes in so does a hormone called prolactin that calms women down and makes them more motherly. (If given to cats it can make them motherly toward mice.) This hormone seems to affect everyone in her environment, perhaps like a pheromone, including siblings and the father. Men seem to be calmer and anxious to help out with the baby when the mother is nursing. She seems more mother-like in her own eyes and those of her friends. She might also be a more calm, kind, considerate person for you to live with. The close physical contact with baby can trigger the outflow of true selfless compassion for all humanity. The intermittent peaceful moments during the day when she must sit down and hold her baby, give her body rest, and her soul peace.

BEST FOOD FOR BABY

What about the baby? From a strict nutritional standpoint, cow's milk can be supplemented with vitamins and additives until it seems to contain all the chemicals necessary for growth. However, there's more to it than chemicals. The protein and other ingredients in milk seem to be specific for each species of animal. Cow's milk was designed for calves, human milk for human babies. When the species are crossed, allergic reactions sometimes develop from "foreign" protein ingestion.

Breast-fed babies are known to grow better, have fewer infections, have less colic, and be more content than the ones on the fanciest cow-milk formula yet devised. Why? For biological *and* psychological reasons. Every time the baby suckles at the breast it signals the mother's body what nutrients and antibodies she needs to produce for the next feeding. Even the U.S. government sponsored an advertising campaign to teach everybody that "Babies Were Born to be Breast Fed." Mothers' milk is best!

BONDING

When a mother holds her baby against the warmth of her skin it reproduces that 98.6-degree body warmth known before. The smooth softness of the breast is similar in touch sensation to the lining of the uterus. Watch the baby fondle and caress the breast during feeding. The fragrance of Mother's skin oils is pleasing to his nostrils. Is this how calves so accurately select their own mothers in a herd of similar-looking cows?

HOME AGAIN

Perhaps the individual protein content of her milk tells his taste buds he's home again. It's hard to test these particular senses—temperature, touch, and smell—in human babies scientifically and objectively. The importance of temperature and touch in the recognition and acceptance of Mother was scientifically demonstrated by the brilliant work of Dr. Harry F. Harlow ("Affectional Responses in the Infant Monkey," *Science,* volume 130, August 21, 1959, pp. 421–432) in rhesus monkey experiments at the University of Wisconsin.

After isolating baby monkeys from their real monkey mothers, he offered them cleverly devised substitute "mothers." These surrogate mothers were inanimate and doll-like in nature and of varied color, texture, and temperature. The two important physical characteristics that made these substitutes acceptable to the baby monkeys were softness to the touch and warmth. The babies would select the warm, soft ones over the others as their choice of mother figures.

HEARTBEAT

Dr. Lee Salk, the psychologist brother of the inventor of a polio vaccine, Dr. Jonas Salk, used human babies to objectively demonstrate the benefit of one aspect of babies' hearing sense, the mother's heartbeat (L. Salk, "The Effects of the Normal Heartbeat Sound on the Behavior of the Newborn Infant: Implications for Mental Health," World Federation of Mental Health report, 1960).

He divided a hospital nursery into two sections and reproduced the recorded sound of a mother's heartbeat over a speaker in one nursery and not in the other, then studied the effect on the babies. He conclusively verified by experimentation an assumption of ours that we have been describing to our patients for years—that human babies, hearing a mother's heartbeat, are more serene, digest their food better, and even grow better than babies who don't hear a mother's heartbeat.

If you obtain a puppy or kitten while it is quite young and separate it from its mother for the first time, it will cry piteously at night. Put two items in its box and the household will be undisturbed—an electric heating pad and a ticking alarm clock! It isn't Mother, but it seems to do until something better shows up. Put a cheap, loud-ticking clock near your baby if you are temporarily out of the room during nap time and the baby will sleep better. Why? Because during the intrauterine life he became accustomed to the rhythmical sounds of Mother's heart beating.

It hasn't been tested, but still another assumption seems reasonable—the rhythmical breath sounds of the mother's lungs, the soft, swishing sound heard through a doctor's stethoscope, can also be heard by the baby. We call this the "breeze in the trees" sound as heard at night in a mountain cabin. Don't you sleep like a baby there?

BREATHING

During the act of breast-feeding, the rhythmical rise and fall of your wife's chest reproduces for your baby a motion sense similar to that caused by her abdominal breathing during sleep, when your baby was in her uterus. Let's add another motion familiar to a baby—rocking. A keen observer can notice the pregnant state of a woman by the rocking motion of her hips as she walks by. This is a consequence of the softening of her pelvic joints, making them mobile, the effect of hormones from the placenta. This brings up two mother commandments in feeding a newborn.

WARMTH

First, she should hold the baby against the warmth of her body. If she is breast-feeding, this is inescapable, but should be done even if bottle-feeding. Never, never prop a bottle on something, then desert the baby.

MOTION

Second, the two of you should invest in a rocking chair so the mother can rock the baby while he's nursing or Dad can rock him when he's fussy.

VERBALIZE

Let's add a **third** commandment—verbalize! Hum, sing, or talk to him in a singsong manner.

You don't have to be a professional singer, just yourself. Yes, Dad, you can talk, or hum, or sing also. The baby is used to the sound of Mother's voice and yours—he listened to it for nine months in the uterus. As doctors, if we are trying to hear the baby's heartbeat through the fetoscope in the prenatal examinations and the mother starts talking, we hastily remove the instrument from our ears; her voice is transmitted so loudly it is uncomfortable.

One theory of why teenagers prefer and enjoy the loud rhythms of rock-and-roll music and rap is that they are meeting their heaviest challenges at adolescence and like to return temporarily to the security of the womb. As experience produces true self-confidence later, such prominent rhythmic beats will not be necessary. But even lots of mature people like background music and find it restful.

Could it be that being cheated out of these reassuring rhythmical sounds by the predominance of bottle-feeding plays a role in the delayed maturing of some adults?

BREAST-FEEDING BENEFITS FOR HUSBANDS

NOTES FROM BRADLEY CLASS FOUR OF TWELVE. BY JAY HATHAWAY, AAHCC

Dr. Bradley learned decades ago that a husband's support makes a critical improvement in the rates and duration of breast-feeding. Science has spent decades catching up.

A study published in 2004 entitled "Dads as Breastfeeding Advocates" concluded: "Expectant fathers can be influential advocates for breastfeeding, playing a critical role in encouraging a woman to breastfeed her newborn infant." (*American Journal of Obstetrics & Gynecology,* volume 191, 2004, 708–12.)

As an experienced dad to six children, I share a few points I use in Bradley class number four (of twelve). If dads understood the benefits breast-feeding brings to them, they might be even more enthusiastic in their support.

FIVE REASONS YOU (DAD) WANT TO SUPPORT BREAST-FEEDING

1. **Financial.** You won't believe how expensive it is to buy all the "stuff" you need to feed ABM (artificial baby milk) to a

baby. The La Leche League used to say you could save the price of a major appliance. I want you to understand this is a major, major appliance. It is unbelievably expensive to pay for formula, bottles, nipples, the extra doctor's visits, and the extra cleaning fees, etc.

2. **Smell.**   Mother's milk is custom-made for your baby, at your baby's particular age. It is almost completely digested. The formula is a foreign substance lacking in the immunities your baby needs. Formula contains many ingredients that are hard or impossible for your child to utilize, for instance human milk is primarily made of a different kind of protein than formula. Breast-fed babies smell nice, and it is even pleasant for a daddy to change their soiled diapers. The baby who struggles to partially digest an artificial, one-type-serves-all formula produces odors that can be powerful. Pretty soon everything you own smells like pungent baby poop.

3. **Two O'Clock in the Morning.**   Do you know what happens to you, the dad, at two a.m.? Do you know how loud a baby cries at two a.m.? Much louder than at two p.m., I'm sure. When you get to your sixth child (our experience) you will have learned that the baby will be happier being breast-fed and sleeping in a family bed, between Mom and Dad. All three get a better night's sleep. And two a.m. becomes no problem.

4. **Travel.**   A breast-fed baby is easy to travel with. Short trips with Mom and baby (like to get a late-night pizza) are easy—just grab a disposable diaper and you're off. Longer trips, like airplane flights are also easier. Nursing helps your baby's sinuses adapt as the plane climbs and descends. Milk is always easily available. If the mom wears well-planned nursing clothing she can nurse most anywhere, and nobody but Mommy and baby know.

5. **Health.**   Both the long-term and short-term health of mother and baby are improved by breast-feeding. The American Academy of Pediatrics, in an official policy statement in 2005 stated: "Human milk is uniquely superior for infant feeding and is species-specific; all substitute

feeding options differ markedly from it. The breastfed infant is the reference or normative model against which all alternative feeding methods must be measured with regard to growth, health, development, and all other short- and long-term outcomes . . . the AAP firmly adheres to the position that breastfeeding ensures the best possible health as well as the best developmental and psychosocial outcomes for the infant. Enthusiastic support and involvement of pediatricians in the promotion and practice of breastfeeding is essential to the achievement of optimal infant and child health, growth, and development." And breast-feeding protects Mommy against breast cancer, too.

Dr. Bradley was way ahead of science on this issue, it truly isn't nice to fool Mother Nature.

BREAST-FEEDING SUMMARY

Support your wife's decision to breast-feed your baby. She may want to regularly attend La Leche League meetings in her neighborhood. Support your wife in kind, subtle ways as well as in verbal ones. Defend her from the criticism of uneducated, inconsiderate, or insensitive people. If in the rare instance she cannot breast-feed for some reason or other, all is not lost. She will still be able to hold the baby, rock him, caress him, talk or sing to him while he is eating.

I could list hundreds of benefits to breast-feeding such as: improved palate, dental, and gum development; benefits of colostrum in terms of antibodies; low cost (this will appeal to coaches); ease to transport; and more. If you want a more complete list, ask a La Leche League leader, a breast-feeding mom, or your Bradley teacher.

13

THE NATURE OF INSTINCT

Natural-childbirth concepts are based upon the principle that human beings are not instinctive animals and must be taught to tune in to their bodies and do what lower animals automatically do by instinct and observing others of their own kind, without training. As we have stressed before, this difference between human beings and other animals is obvious in their respective conduct in water and in labor.

However, anyone contemplating this theory would reflect on some instances in which human behavior under the stress of childbirth or in keeping afloat in water seemed to demonstrate instinctive, automatic behavior—without preliminary training. Indeed, Dr. Grantly Dick-Read, a British pioneer in natural childbirth and author of *Childbirth without Fear* (Heinemann Medical Books, 1942), was first inspired by the calm, instinctive conduct of a mother who smilingly turned down his offer of gas because, she said, "God didn't intend it to hurt."

Any medical personnel associated with obstetrics very long will be impressed by the variety of conduct of different women in labor. Not all untrained mothers in labor panic, scream, and ask to be "knocked out" and "delivered." I can use the example of my own six-foot-tall, deeply religious, English Canadian mother who not only calmly gave unmedicated birth to eleven pounds of me, but kidded the attending doctor because he perspired and she didn't.

Could it be possible that, after all, human beings do have instinctive powers?

Let's consider the human brain and its function and "brainstorm" a bit about this elusive ability known as instinct. Could it possibly be that human brains do share this ability with other animals but that somewhere in the evolutionary development of more complex brains we have lost the ability to use it in most instances?

In the anatomic examination of the human brain we find an "older" portion that resembles that of the lower animals. The outer covering or cortex of the human brain, which presumably evolved more recently, is much thicker and more complex than that of the lower animals. This is the portion that is thought to function in abstract thinking and reasoning. In human beings it is highly developed.

With all this superior equipment, why do we humans have to be "delivered" of our young as if they were something evil and abnormal? Or do we? Not in some instances. Why the difference? If as a Bradley labor coach you are to be effective, you must be convincing. In order to be convincing to your wife you must first be convinced in your own mind. Toward that end let's consider the function of human brains. Brevity dictates oversimplification, but your relationship to your wife and to your child depends upon insight into these functions.

In my opinion, human brains do have full instinctive abilities, just like those of the lower animals. For convenience we think of these abilities as being housed and functioning in the inner, older "animal" part of our brain. For simplicity we will refer to this area as governing the subconscious.

Why do only some human beings under some conditions sometimes manifest instinct? If it's so beneficial, why do not all people use it at all times? Because it is not always available for use. The cortex of human brains can, because of its very complexity, act as a cover-up to the underlying animal brain.

This outer layer, for convenience, we will refer to as controlling the conscious mind of man. These two functions are not mutually exclusive, the conscious and the subconscious. Rather they are constantly interacting and affecting each other. The more complicated the conscious mind has become, the more it interferes with instinctive abilities. For instance, prior to the age of six months, human infants manifest swimming instinct; they either swim automatically or are very easy to teach. After six months the conscious cover-up begins to form. Learning responsibility results in development of fear, anxiety, and worry, which interferes with instinctive conduct.

Could the religious convictions of my mother and Dr. Dick-Read's patient have caused a serenity that thinned the clouds of anxiety and fear, allowing the automatic guidance of instinct to penetrate? As an obstetrician, I have seen this many times.

Can prenatal education and guidance coupled with the reassuring presence of the man she loves, constantly coaching and encouraging, allow your wife to function as an instinctive animal, enabling her to joyously give birth? Yes, indeed, I have seen this many, many times, too.

Why are some women so much easier to teach to give birth than others? Let's answer that by substituting for convenience the instinctive function, swimming, for that of birth. Why are some human beings so much easier to teach to swim than others? Could the individual who "takes to water like a duck" possess a thinner conscious cloud layer than the difficult pupil whose cloud layer was thickened by fear of water due to some unpleasant previous experience or, perhaps, fear following gruesome suggestions planted previously by thoughtless people?

Even the most frightened conscious-clouded human being can, by patient instruction and reassurance, overcome fear and anxiety and be taught to swim. The same applies to your wife and childbirth. Barring physical abnormalities, there is no woman who can't by patient instruction be taught to give birth.

These are only two manifestations of instinct. To understand its nature further, what instinctive functions other than swimming and birth might be manifested by human beings? Are these others also applicable to our lives? Instinct has been recognized for many centuries, although the exact nature of it and how it works has not as yet been determined. It is about time we quit ignoring the irrefutable fact that it works and turn the academic light of science upon it for a more thorough study. The possibility that human beings may share instinctive abilities with animals has awakened some interest. Increasing evidence that supports this possibility is being brought to light. We have much to gain in better interpersonal relations by more extensive studies in this area.

Telepathy falls within the category of human instincts. What does recognizing the telepathic ability of some human beings have to do with your life, your wife, your baby? More than you perhaps realize. Babies and young children have thin conscious-cloud layers due to inexperience and dependence. Their little telepathic receivers function very efficiently. An article in a popular magazine featured brain-wave tracing of a mother and her infant taken all night long during sleep. It was observed that the pattern of pleasant dreaming and unpleasant, disturbed dreaming was identical for both mother and child. In other words, the baby, even while asleep, sensed each time its mother was disturbed. When its mother was serene, so was the baby. Was this an objective measurement of human instinctual telepathy?

Our breast-feeding mothers tell me about a game they play when away from their older babies. They have the babysitter record the exact time the baby cries to be fed. Meantime, the mother records the exact time her breasts have the "let-down" feeling. In comparing the times, they are identical! Apply this to other human relationships. What are the practical aspects of awareness of such human communicability? Plenty! Thoughts run through my mind of that young couple who have a baby to "hold their marriage together." They sweet-talk each other in front of the child while harboring hostility toward each other in their subconscious "animal" minds—and wonder why the child becomes a nervous, neurotic, insecure individual. He senses that hostility telepathically. Don't try to kid kids!

Another disturbing memory comes to my mind: PTA meetings where I have met frustrated women who are teaching elementary school but who do not like children. Their syrupy sweet talk before the class goes for naught. These children sense that subconscious dislike and react with hostility. How much better children perform and what inspiration they receive when a compassionate teacher who truly loves children is guiding them subconsciously.

Clairvoyance is another category of instinct. Is there a "mind's eye" at this level that can see, even at great distances and in spite of physical obstacles? This is evidenced in animals' homing instinct, the sore-footed cat or dog that returns home no matter where it's taken.

Why can't we lose them? They seem to be able to "see" home, even an empty house when no one is there. (If some person or animal is present at home, this would complicate the picture by the possibility of its being telepathic perception.) This was dramatically illustrated in Walt Disney's film *The Incredible Journey*, relating the ability of two dogs and a cat to return to an empty home over great distances and in spite of many obstacles in their path.

Can human minds do this? There is much evidence that they can. A high percentage of similar phenomena occur in interpersonal relationships of mother love and other close emotional ties, as when a mother "sees" the exact scene of an accident involving her child.

To illustrate the current interest in instinct and animal brain function: As I was writing this chapter an advertisement appeared in a national magazine picturing a dolphin coming up out of a pool of water to speak into a microphone that was connected with an electronic computer designed to translate Dolphinese automatically into English. The computer company was very serious. Interspecies communication is not only possible but is probable in the near future.

The era we are now living in may be recorded by the historians of tomorrow as the "space age." However, they will be referring not only to outer space, but also to the increased utilization of that elusive animal portion of our brains that performs instinctively—inner space.

Your function as a parent and as a companion to your wife is intimately related to your recognition of these basic forms of interpersonal instinctual means of communication. Your inner peace of mind, your sincere deep thoughts of love and affection, will be received telepathically by your wife and child.

The closer the emotional ties, the more perceptive the subconscious mind. This is the basic reason why you, as a lover and husband, make the ideal labor coach and companion. Your wife really feels close to you. Your calmness and confidence will be imparted to her and utilized efficiently to meet the stress of labor. There is no adequate substitute for the husband.

14

RESEARCH CATCHES UP WITH
THE BRADLEY METHOD

Publishers like to revise an existing book about every seven years, bringing it up to date to fit new research.

I'm proud to state that this is not necessary for our method; rather, the reverse is true. Modern research is finally being brought up to date, simply verifying the truth of every principle we stood for originally. Research is justifying our method, not vice versa. Let's illustrate with a few examples.

The Bradley Method is very flattered by the Johnny-come-lately methods that imitate the great principles we originated, advocated, and have used since 1947, then proclaim them to be original with the newcomers. For example: walking about ("putsy-putsy" phase) in early labor; gentle deep abdominal breathing rather than hyperventilation (we have never had our patients put paper sacks over their heads to rebreathe CO_2 as some of the other methods advocate); total and complete abstention from drugs wherever possible (one method even taught drug use in prenatal classes, then reversed to our concepts when enormous amounts of research verified our approach).

HUSBAND-COACH

The use of husbands as labor coaches (instead of female "monitrices, doulas, labor companions, or labor assistants"), which I first introduced in 1947, has been adopted by others. Some had the audacity to claim this was original with them years after I had advocated it.

BREAST-FEEDING

Also, the immediate breast-feeding of babies at birth is something "new," although we have taught it all these years as natural. Allowing mothers to go home from the hospital as soon as two hours after birth to escape separation from their babies in the newborn nursery, is not new. Going home early is a "now" fad we have been practicing all these many years. So research has finally caught up with The Bradley Method. Where were these new authorities in 1947?

THE IV

Another no-no we have stressed as unnatural is the routine IV glucose given mothers in labor. I didn't know why this shouldn't be done, but all these years have pointed out that as mother animals out in the woods don't need IV glucose, neither should human mothers, unless, of course, they are ill. New research demonstrated this "why" very skillfully.

The increased glucose in the maternal circulation goes directly through the placenta to the infant. The baby responds with high insulin output to counteract it, then when it is born, the maternal glucose suddenly ceases and the baby is left with extra insulin, resulting in hypoglycemia, or low blood sugar. It's truly not wise to fool Mother Nature.

IATROGENIC (DOCTOR-CAUSED) PREMATURITY

New research verifies the ill effects of inducing labor artificially, with its high incidence of respiratory distress and in iatrogenic (doctor-caused) prematurity. Only God knows when a baby is ready to be born, and when that baby is ready, natural labor will ensue. Why must people interfere?

LEAVING THE HOSPITAL

Leaving the hospital early with naturally born babies also makes sense in view of the steadily rising incidence of hospital-resistant bacterial infections. Our theory is that a hospital is sometimes the proper place to bear a child, but the most dangerous place to board one. This has been verified by research.

INCUBATOR

The old idea that a newborn had to be placed—just to keep warm—in an incubator or hot box at birth instead of experiencing its mother's arms and breasts has also been researched and found ridiculous in unmedicated mothers and babies. The infants do not get cold next to their mother's skin with a warm blanket over both—which has always seemed so logical. Beanies (little hats) are used to conceal obstetric injuries, not really to heat the baby's head. Some loss of heat from the baby's head is normal. Babies have survived over millions of years without their beanies.

LONG-TERM BREAST-FEEDING

The many benefits of immediate and long-term breast-feeding of infants has even got the seal of approval of the pediatricians, finally. What could be more obvious?

SMOKING AND ALCOHOL

The ill effects of smoking and of ingesting alcohol in pregnancy are now front-page news. I've been warning women about these drugs for half a century. My file of research on these principles bulges with articles verifying what we have assumed for so long.

ULTRASOUND INACCURATE AND POSSIBLY DANGEROUS

I am concerned about both the safety and accuracy of ultrasound. Parents should be cautious and use ultrasound only when necessary for a valid medical reason. I am outraged at parents paying for ultrasound "keepsake videos" as home movies just for fun. I stopped counting the number of times couples have been told the wrong sex, due date, or weight of their baby.

Ultrasound has been wrong over and over again, even about twins and deformities. The use of ultrasound is appropriate on some occasions, but the National Institutes of Health says, ". . . up to $1 billion could be saved each year if ultrasound examinations were limited to high-risk pregnancies or when problems arise" (NICHD, press release, September 15, 1993).

An official government publication, the *FDA Consumer* (January–February 2004, as well as an earlier article in 1994), warned: Ultrasound energy delivered to the fetus cannot be regarded as innocuous. The Department of Health and Human Services has released another information bulletin stating, "Persons who promote, sell or lease ultrasound equipment for making 'keepsake' fetal videos should know that we view this as an unapproved use of medical equipment." FDA officials have said that ultrasound can generate heat in fetal tissue, create microscopic bubbles and cause vibrations, all of which might affect fetal development. As with any technology, carefully weigh the risks versus the benefits.

Physical therapists and chiropractors refuse to use ultrasound on growth areas of children's bones. Could this be a problem for developing fetuses? Is there a problem exposing fetuses' ovaries to ultrasound? Lots of questions—only time will tell.

HAPPINESS, DIGNITY, AND PRIDE

Last but not least, the happiness, dignity, and pride in personal accomplishment that so many years ago prompted me to have the husband there to share has been shown to bond fathers to babies and to their wives, with a lowering of divorce rates, child abuse incidence, etc., as well as those beautiful, healthy Bradley babies. It is truly God's method, the way He taught it to animals via inner instinctive drives, and the way we human beings must learn to do it by imitation. When we do perform this method, the babies and the parents are truly blessed.

UPDATED EVIDENCE

CESAREAN EPIDEMIC

The most recent data available as of this revision, released by the Centers for Disease Control and the National Center for Health Statistics in December 2007, shows an amazing 31.1 percent of all births were cesareans. They admit the rate has risen 50 percent since 1996.

HARM FROM CESAREAN

There are many harmful aspects to using major abdominal surgery to replace labor and birth. One example: A study released in 2005 in the *American Journal of Obstetrics & Gynecology* linked cesarean to breathing problems in babies. To quote: "Cesarean delivery was an independent risk factor for RDS (Respiratory Distress Syndrome). The risk was reduced with labor before a cesarean but still elevated."

INDUCING LABOR

The *Journal of Reproductive Medicine* in 2002 was headlined by Reuters: "Induced Labor Rate in US More Than Doubled in a Decade." They predicted a 30 percent rate by 2007. Why, have women changed? Or have their doctors?

INDUCTION DRUG DANGER

The U.S. Food and Drug Administration released, in 2005, an "FDA Alert" regarding the drug misoprostol (marketed as

Cytotec). They admitted this drug is currently being used to "begin labor." They report: "There can be serious side effects . . . [including] the death of the mother or baby." The alert clearly states, "These uses are not approved by the FDA."

DRUGS IN LABOR

The journal *Epidemiology* in 2000 showed a link between drugs used in birthing, and adult drug abuse in the babies when they grew up. Reporting on this finding Reuters Health reported: "Women who wish to lower their offspring's risk of drug abuse may decide to forego some of their own drug use during labor and delivery."

ELECTRONIC FETAL MONITORING

The *American Journal of Obstetrics & Gynecology* in 2000 asked the question; "Fetal heart rate monitoring: Is it salvageable?" and even asked ". . . whether fetal heart rate monitoring should be abandoned." The American College of Obstetricians and Gynecologists advised the obstetricians of America in 2005: "Given that the available data do not clearly support EFM over intermittent auscultation (using a stethoscope), either option is acceptable in a patient without complications." The British journal *Lancet* said EFM is "a widespread and expensive practice that is largely unjustified."

ULTRASOUND

Ultrasound has become nearly universal, but without proof of safety. It is used for scans, external EFM, even those little electronic stethoscopes (doptones). There are many studies that raise important questions. In July 1993 the *British Medical Journal* reported, "The odds of non-right handedness were higher among children who had been scanned." Then, in November 2003, the *Journal of the Canadian Medical Association* found an association between prenatal ultrasonography and delayed speech. These sound trivial, but what else don't we yet know? How does ultrasound radiation affect speech or handedness? The American College of Obstetricians and Gynecologists officially says, "Ultrasound should be performed only when there is a valid medical indication, and the lowest possible ultrasonic exposure setting should be used."

In August 2006 a study done at the Yale University School of Medicine suggested that ". . . ultrasound can affect the development of the fetal brain. . . . When pregnant mice were exposed to ultrasound, a small number of nerve cells in the developing brains of their fetuses failed to extend correctly in the cerebral cortex."

EPISIOTOMY

For decades there have been studies that questioned its value. Then, in 2005, the *Journal of the American Medical Association* said, "Evidence does not support maternal benefits . . . outcomes with episiotomy can be considered worse."

BREAST-FEEDING MOTHERS AND BABIES

Yale University researchers in 2001, quoted by the Associated Press, found: "Women who breast-fed their babies for two years or longer reduced their risk of breast cancer by 50 percent." In 2005, the American Academy of Pediatrics issued a "Policy Statement" supporting what Dr. Bradley had taught and advocated since 1947: "Human milk is uniquely superior."

15

OBSTACLES TO OVERCOME

OBSTACLE ONE: THE MEDICAL PROFESSION

A steadily increasing group of doctors is advocating The Bradley Method of natural childbirth and an active rather than passive role for the husband. However, there are still a few doctors against this concept. Why? Many reasons. I think the first and most important is that they have never truly tried it. This is obvious in some of the statements made by the most clamorous opponents. If the old adage "Don't knock it if you haven't tried it" were properly applied, there would be no further opposition.

Another excuse expressed is that doctors haven't the time to use it. This was refuted by statistical studies revealing the shortening of labor, the decreased number of doctors' examinations needed, and so forth, when trained husbands are coaching (R. A. Bradley, "Father's Presence in Delivery Rooms," *Psychosomatics,* volume 3, number 6, 1962).

The American Academy of Husband-Coached Childbirth, The Bradley Method regularly trains and certifies childbirth educators. I had the privilege of helping to train these teachers and was delighted by the feedback received at our meetings of the Academy on how doctors are enthusiastically using their services. Our teachers give the doctor a well-trained couple, who know what they are doing, and who by their gratitude and enthusiasm greatly enhance his practice as well as save his time.

Our teachers are nearly all experienced unmedicated mothers and all have taken the intensive training course and examination for certification by our Academy. The executive directors and founders of the Academy are an enthusiastic couple, Jay and Marjie Hathaway, who have done more to make childbirth safe and joyful than anyone I know.

They have had six babies themselves—the first three were outmoded medicated deliveries. With number four, they had heard about our program in Denver and, as they couldn't get it in California, they flew to Denver with Marjie in labor and joyfully gave birth, husband coaching, no drugs or medication, breast-fed on the table at birth, walked back—the whole works. Today their son James is executive vice president of our Academy.

I verbally chastised them both for flying here in labor, and then told them to go home and change their outmoded hospitals and doctors. To my surprise, they did just that!

Thanks to their dedicated work, the state of California leads all others in husband-coached natural childbirth, which the Hathaways insisted upon calling "The Bradley Method." They made a marvelous movie, *Childbirth for the Joy of It,* showing several women giving birth, ecstatically, to their first babies, without thoughts of drugs. They had a fifth child by our method in California; little Robert weighed almost ten pounds, and as I had weighed eleven pounds at birth, he was named, I'm proud to state, after me. Robert was followed by another unmedicated, spontaneously born, immediately breast-fed, bright, active youngster. This one, a little girl, was named Ann and is a charmer.

Anyone who has experienced husband-coached natural childbirth and would like to take the intensive training course to become a teacher should contact the Academy (1-800-4-A-BIRTH, www.bradleybirth.com). Husbands and wives are preferred teaching as a team, but experienced Bradley moms can also teach. If there are no teachers of The Bradley Method of true natural childbirth in your area, consider being a pioneer teacher. Your hospitals, doctors, and parents will be forever grateful.

One would think that if a woman expressed a desire to give birth to her offspring actively and unassisted and found the act such a happy, joyful experience that she would like to share it with her husband, the very least the medical profession could do would be to cooperate with her. On the surface, this seems a simple request. In my personal experience, doctors are very much needed by about 3 percent of our patients, to do life-saving cesarean sections. They are also needed by another 3 percent who, for various reasons, require to be delivered or medicated in birth. Of the remaining 94 percent, after careful prenatal training, the role of the doctor at the moment of birth is so insignificant as to be almost belittling, most of the time we doctors should merely be lifeguards, and be there for support and medical backup. We take a lot of kidding from our patients regarding this. "What am I paying you for? I did all the work!"

But they are expressing pride in their own accomplishment and not really criticizing. They realize that the most important work of their doctor is to stand by in case of unforeseen complications.

We advocates of natural childbirth point out that the primary duty of a doctor is the prenatal inspiration of a patient and her husband to want to work together to give spontaneous birth. Most training centers teach budding doctors only the mechanics of abnormal obstetrics and ignore the psychological management of normal obstetrics. Pregnant women should be looked upon not just as baby factories but as complex human beings with a mind, a soul, and a body.

Another obstacle to acceptance by the medical profession is that the method represents a taboo-breaking innovation. The history of medicine reveals a reluctance to change accepted established techniques. The old taboo that a husband does not belong at the scene of birth, the old taboo that there is a magical halo about the attending physician that would be diminished or destroyed by the presence of the participating husband, and the oldest of all taboos, generating from the mistranslation of Genesis (H. Wessel, *Natural Childbirth and the Family*, New York: Harper & Row, 1974) that a baby's birth should be attended with pain and sorrow—all of these taboos are torn asunder by modern concepts of natural childbirth. This is a mighty big pill for the medical profession to swallow quickly at one gulp. It takes time.

Remember the words of Max Planck. As a layperson don't try to educate established older physicians to your way of thinking even if you sincerely feel you're right and they are wrong. Rather, keep looking until you find an already educated doctor, usually a younger one.

Most doctors are egocentric. This is nearly a necessity in the practice of medicine for psychological reasons. Most doctors in established practice bitterly resent laypeople teaching them another way of doing obstetrics. You are insulting them by implying that what they are doing and have been doing for years is wrong and your way is right.

A teenage mother, daughter of an established doctor, tells how she had to have her third child by natural childbirth (unmedicated, joyful, walking back from the delivery room, going home in two hours, etc.) before her physician father changed his resentful attitude and grudgingly admitted that maybe there was something to the method, after all.

For you, the proper approach is to patronize the doctor who thinks and acts in accordance with these principles. Don't accept a patient-hungry doctor who will "go along" with you, but keep looking until you find one who shares your interest, one who will teach and encourage you. I recall one couple who had visited, and hurriedly left, seventeen doctors before they found what they wanted. I can think of no greater stimulus to a doctor to investigate natural childbirth than to have his office door shut with great vigor several times by hurriedly departing patients.

Today many magazine articles, especially in *Mothering Magazine* (www.mothering.com), are written on the dangers of giving anesthetics to mothers, the ill effects of medication for the new-born, and the psychological and spiritual importance of prenatal education for both husband and wife. Often these articles also stress the need of special physical training to properly perform an athletic physical event like giving birth. Experienced parents write about the rich emotional rewards of conscious birth-time again and again in lay magazines.

With natural childbirth used and the husband present, the mother and father are two interested, analytical observers. Some doctors are uncomfortable under such observation. They don't like to be watched in their work. Such an attitude reflects a lack of self-confidence. Keep looking until you find a doctor who is self-confident and takes pride in being observed.

If you are fortunate enough to have a natural-childbirth teacher in your area trained and certified by the American Academy of Husband-Coached Childbirth, simply ask for the teacher's suggestions on which doctor and hospital to attend. They know by experience which ones follow these principles.

OBSTACLE TWO: YOUR PARENTS

Some women are thrilled their daughters give birth naturally when they didn't, but for others it may be very irritating to have suffered a long, gruesome labor, to have been sickened with anesthesia, to have felt she suffered the agony of the damned, to have been hospitalized for days, even weeks, bringing a girl child into the world—then to have her daughter grow up, marry, get pregnant, and nonchalantly give birth without medication, walk back from the birth room, go home two hours later, and then add insult to injury by enthusiastically raving about how much fun it all was.

I had such a woman call me in fury one night. She claimed hysterically that I had turned her child against her! I ought to be ashamed! I couldn't figure out what on earth she was talking about at first. The story finally came out. Her daughter had happily given birth by natural-childbirth principles, left the hospital in two hours, and headed straight for her mother's house. When her mother answered the door the daughter shook her mother until her teeth rattled and verbally hurt her even worse. "I hate you, I hate you. All my life you held over me how you suffered having me. You lied. I just had a baby and it didn't hurt a bit!"

I became a wiser individual that night, and from then on incorporated the admonition into our prenatal training—don't hold it against your mother if she had a terrible time bearing you; she isn't fibbing. Bear in mind it wasn't her fault. She didn't have the benefit in those days of careful mental and physical preparation for birth. She was not attended constantly by a trained, love-motivated coach, her husband.

Fathers of our patients are also an obstacle occasionally. They subconsciously recall the indignity of their useless, separated, guilt-ridden role and unwittingly resent the useful participating role of modern husbands. Such unconscious resentment can be alleviated in most parents by having them attend classes or read the same material with you. "It's so different now," I've heard from their lips so many times. Indeed, thank God, it is different now.

OBSTACLE THREE: YOUR FRIENDS

"I told my doctor: 'Just give me drugs.' " How many times have you heard that sentiment or something like it from your female friends? "Forget natural childbirth. Just knock me out." Many women are not really interested in childbirth or in hard work, and take refuge in looking down on those who are. They are, of course, entitled to their opinion. Don't get into any heated arguments; their rigid minds are frozen in self-defense. They are to be pitied, not argued with.

As I have often said, the greatest handicap in practicing this type of obstetrics is the overenthusiasm of the patients and their husbands. They often tend to make a distinct nuisance of themselves.

One new obstetrical couple presented themselves in late

pregnancy. I mistakenly thought this was their first visit to the doctor and began the conversation with a critical question to this effect. The lady snapped at me defensively, "I've been going to another doctor regularly!" I looked bewildered and asked why they wanted to change so late in pregnancy.

She looked dejected and frustrated and rather pointedly explained, "Well, we bought a new house. Our next-door neighbor turned out to be one of your natural-childbirth mothers. She told me that if I didn't have enough respect for my own children to learn how to give birth to them she'd never speak to me again! We have to live next to her, so here I am! We like our new house." She and her husband became wonderful, cooperative patients, but I had to start with an apology for the enthusiasm of their neighbors.

OBSTACLE FOUR: HOSPITAL PERSONNEL

Some years ago I received a letter from a mom who said:

> Hospitals are distinctly unpleasant places to me in that they are too often operated by personnel who have no regard for human dignity; this at least has been my experience with hospitals; I sincerely hope that my own experiences have been exceptional, and that not all women are treated as I have been. Most registered cows receive more considerate treatment when they have calves than I received on the three occasions when I had babies in a hospital.

Hospitals are very good places to be, of course, when one is really sick. This is because they are geared to the needs of sick people. But a woman undergoing a normal delivery without fear is not sick, and is therefore somewhat out of place in the average hospital, unless she can adjust to the idea of being treated as if she were sick.

If you are in a hospital that is relatively unacquainted with natural childbirth, the staff may be skeptical of you. It seems ridiculous, but it's true. I have seen some attending nurses, even interns, and especially anesthetists who by their facial expressions and attitudes show they resent a mother giving birth without their medication. Don't worry about it. Ignore them. Mind your own business so well that they can't help eventually admiring you.

A few hospitals benefit from nurses and attendants trained and experienced in natural childbirth. If you are a pioneer, take personal pride in it and don't resent an occasional slight.

As times continue to change, hospitals that keep a husband and wife together in labor will be doing a booming business, and the ones that separate them will be losing business. This is becoming evident already. Don't waste your time with the inexperienced and the prejudiced while you are preparing for the birth of your baby. If you or your wife encounter obstacles that are bothersome, discuss them with your Bradley teacher, other natural-childbirth couples, and supportive medical professionals. I admire those who, even in the face of opposition, have the courage of their convictions and the intestinal fortitude to practice accordingly.

After your baby's birth write letters to people who were stumbling blocks to let them know you did it, that natural childbirth works. Relate your positive experience and share your joy. A thank-you letter to those who dared to help and support you also may make a difference.

16

PREGNANCY LOSS

Nature is not noted for efficiency when it comes to reproducing species in all animals and insects. In order to get a good living representative of the species, many babies are lost along the way. We do not know why, but this applies equally to human beings as to all other species. Losses can occur early as well as late in pregnancy. Perhaps it is nature's quality control system.

"WHAT IF MY WIFE HAS A MISCARRIAGE?"

There are many possible causes for early pregnancies ending in spontaneous miscarriages. By far the most frequent cause is the simple fact that your wife was developing pregnancy signs without a baby or with only parts of a baby being present. This could just as easily result from nonviable sperm or eggs. Even in the healthiest, most robust men there is a certain percentage of abnormal sperm present in the semen. This is a "normal abnormality," which occurs in all other animal species as well as the human.

For years I have been directing my patients to ignore the old "bad egg," blighted-ovum theory of the cause of miscarriages. I based my argument on statistics that about one in five sperm in healthy young men have chromosomal abnormalities and that about one in four to five pregnancies miscarry, in all species of mammals, including the human. I get irritated over blaming everything on women.

As a farm boy, I noted that stud fee receipts for getting our mare pregnant guaranteed a "standing colt." If a miscarriage occurred, they brought the mare back to the same stud horse for another try—they didn't get another mare!

Our French poodle miscarried her first pregnancy, then proceeded to litter the place with seven healthy pups on her next pregnancy—same father, too. On the farm, horses, cows, pigs, and so forth, also have miscarriages. They pass empty amniotic sacs or sacs containing only fragments of fetal material instead of a complete fetus.

It is true that there are some women who lose good babies, but this is very rare, and when it happens your doctor will investigate for possible causes. If you see a mother with five children, she's probably had one or more early miscarriages. It is true that some women have twelve pregnancies and no miscarriages, but it seems to be on a purely chance basis; enough other women have miscarriages to keep the percentage about constant when a large sample is studied.

It is hard to estimate the actual number, as many women have a late, crampy menstrual period and never recognize it as a miscarriage or bother to report it to a doctor. Most miscarriages occur around the second or third missed period time, some earlier, some later.

What could your wife do to prevent such a possibility from happening?

Nothing. There's nothing known that she does, or doesn't do, that will alter the incidence. Grandmother was put to bed—and had just as many miscarriages there as being up and around. Many a woman harbors a guilt complex because she attributes something she did just before she miscarried as the cause. These "somethings" would fill three volumes—lifting, riding in a car, intercourse, travel, worry, fright—and have no known relationship to the miscarriage except sequence. What follows is not necessarily due to what preceded. Just because more gray-haired men have heart attacks than non-gray-haired men doesn't mean we can conclude that gray hair causes attacks.

Do not let your wife blame herself for a miscarriage. Remember our examples of out-of-wedlock women who try everything on earth short of internal manipulations to destroy the baby, but fail.

The other way around is applicable, too. If your wife has a pregnancy with placenta and amniotic sac present but no fetus in the sac, she will have a miscarriage come hell or high water, no matter what she does. From the medical standpoint, doctors treat all threatening miscarriages as if good babies were present, for the simple reason that until the amniotic sac comes out, no one knows. Even ultrasound may be wrong.

The general rule is applicable: If a good baby is present, it will stay put and grow, even with irregular bleeding and/or cramps. If a good baby isn't present, the wise uterus will empty itself and try again later. Ultrasound may give some clues to this, but may also put the baby at risk at the same time.

Some uteri need a little help emptying themselves and your doctor may choose to do a D & C. This dilatation and curettage of the uterus consists in stretching or dilating the cervix to allow the entrance of a curette. This instrument is like a long iced-tea spoon with sharp edges. It is used to scrape, cleanse, and remove the nonviable material in the uterus. (There is also a new suction-type curette that removes the material by negative pressure.) This cuts down on the loss of blood the uterus would probably have used to cleanse itself of nonviable material. If a woman passes all the material and does not bleed to excess doing it—and this is the normal course in over 95 percent of miscarriages—there is no need to do anything except get pregnant again, and better luck next time.

Luck or chance, not management, will determine whether a good sperm fertilizes a good egg. And ignore your grandmother's

"If only you hadn't done such and such." When you have a good sperm with a good egg, the baby will remain and grow to maturity, regardless of what you do or don't do. A miscarriage is Mother Nature's quality control system.

"WHAT IF MY WIFE HAS A STILLBORN BABY?"

One of our Doberman pinscher dogs gave birth to a litter of seven pups. Although the mother dog was only one year old, you would have thought she had read this book and been to our classes, for she calmly did everything right, just the way it is described here. However, out of seven puppies we only had six living, as one had died before birth. In nearly all species of animals there is the occasional dead baby from unmanageable and unforeseeable intrauterine complications.

With all our scientific advances in obstetrics, we still get the occasional human stillbirth. Sheer chance plays a role; we have no way of controlling or predicting it. We try to detect cord problems by electronic fetal monitoring, but it doesn't seem any more efficient than listening to the fetal heart by stethoscope.

By the time we realize something is wrong, it is frequently too late. In other extremely rare cases everything seems normal, then on the final passage, the baby can die just before it is born. It could be from an unsuspected nuchal (around the neck) cord being drawn tight by the infant's descent. Nuchal cords are common; harm from them is rare, indeed. Another rare cause could be the placenta separating early, causing excessive bleeding, which can be an immediate threat of death to the baby. There can be other causes, as well.

A stillbirth is very upsetting to the parents, the doctor, and the attendants, but in spite of all precautions it is bound to occur occasionally. We offer sincere sympathy, as doctors, to the grieving parents. I recommend you contact your Bradley teacher for local resources.

The old adage applies: "If at first you don't succeed, try, try again," and this is the natural pattern we see in all species.

Losing a baby is never a pleasant event, and some couples have found the book *Empty Cradle, Broken Heart,* by Deborah Davis, Ph.D. (Fulcrum Publishing, 1996), shares some helpful information. Perhaps one of the most amazing things is the resilience of the human infant. Hundreds of thousands of babies are born each and every day.

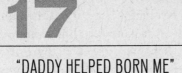

17

"DADDY HELPED BORN ME"

With yesterday's unprepared mothers and medicated methods of childbirth, husbands were mercifully excluded from the delivery room, and the idea of taking a picture of the mother and child at the moment of birth was even more unheard of and horrible to contemplate.

However, with today's prepared mothers and ever-present husbands the birth of a baby and the radiant, joyful look on an unmedicated mother's face at the moment she first sees and holds her child are something to be remembered always, via photographs, rather than something to be forgotten, via anesthetics.

Accordingly, under two courageous administrators of Porter Memorial Hospital in Denver, Colorado, Olof T. Moline and, earlier, Harley E. Rice, husbands were not only allowed to be present but were permitted to bring cameras and record this important moment. These most precious of pictures, as one couple referred to them, have come to be known as "daddy pictures" and are proudly placed on page one of the baby book.

Grateful husbands have given us copies, which have now accumulated into hundreds of prints. They are put on display at conventions and gather crowds of enthusiastic people who just can't get over how healthy and happy the mothers look and how pink and vigorous the yelling babies are at the moment of birth.

As an invited lecturer at banquets, I have announced that the audience may now view pictures taken by husbands of their wives and babies at the moment of birth. It is amusing to see the reaction before viewing ("Please, we have just eaten!") compared with the exclamations of wonder and amazement after viewing ("How can she look that good?").

On a rainy day in Denver a little girl brought her toddler friends indoors to look at books. The favorite book she selected to show her playmates was her baby book. Its first pages contained the snapshots taken by her father of her and her mother at the actual moment of birth, as well as other views that included her father, taken by attendants.

Her proud explanatory statement to her playmates as they viewed these pictures together, "Daddy helped born me," was overheard by her mother and related to us. Childishly ungrammatical as it may be, I deem those four words most symbolic of all that this book and my life's work stand for. Consider the first word, **"Daddy."** Daddy felt her birth was such an important personal event that he was there to help her mother perform it. It was such a happy occasion to him that he felt it warranted his taking pictures to preserve the memory of it. These "daddy pictures" constituted something worthy to show to her friends on rainy days.

In the little girl's mind was a feeling of having been wanted by her father as well as her mother—a feeling of having by her very entrance into this world made two people very happy and proud. Compare the feelings forever associated in her mind with the anniversary of this wonderful occasion, her birth day, with those associated by a child who inadvertently overheard her mother bitterly condemn her delivery day as a most horrible experience: "Never again. That d— man can have the next one!"

What effect does all this have on the mind and soul of a child? Compare the paternal effect of the man who states he always gets drunk at the local bar while his wife is being delivered and the effect of the man who maintains to all who will listen that the most meaningful moment of his life was being present at the birth of his child.

How much closer is the father-child relationship when he can truly say, "I was there when you were born—and I have pictures to prove it." It is heartwarming to find how many fathers carry copies of their pictures in their wallets and how eagerly they display them.

Note the little girl's second word, "**helped.**" Daddy wasn't an idle visitor or a mere curiosity seeker. The concept that husbands help, that childbirth is a shared experience, was recognized in that child's mind at such a tender age. What a wonderful mother she will grow up to be.

This little girl and others like her won't mature to resent their own femininity and bitterly condemn the passive role of their husbands. Their philosophy will not be, "If men had to bear children, there wouldn't be any!" Their obstetrician will have little to do. They'll be wonderful mothers.

The third word, "**born,**" ungrammatical as it may be, denoted to that child that her mother did something to bring her into the world. The mother was not possessed of something evil from which she should be "delivered." She was possessed of something that was nice—me. She was pregnant, a state of "preparing to bring forth."

God did not intend babies as an idle gift from a "delivery service," but as a rich reward for a mother's effort in bringing forth. I recently visited a hospital where the intensive-care division of obstetrics had the usual label, "Delivery Room," on the door. However, in the adjoining section for natural childbirth, the birth rooms were labeled, "Borning Rooms." I was delighted.

Even the child's fourth word, "**me,**" has significance. "Me" was the star of this show. All this fuss and bother was for me. I was the central figure for which all the preparation was made, whose arrival was such an important occasion that pictures were taken by my daddy to make a permanent record so that my birth will always be remembered. The awareness of personal identity is contained there.

In my travels lecturing on my beloved method of childbirth, I am envious of the progress made in some hospitals, even more than my own. I have been met at meetings of natural-childbirth parents by little children proudly wearing little T-shirts with the lettering, "My Daddy Helped Born Me" and also by baby-buggy parades with this sign on the buggies.

I have seen hospitals with such good awareness of our principles that video cameras are permanently installed in their birth rooms, with a control button at the doctor's feet, and tapes of the births are presented to the parents. What could be better public relations for the hospital than this? How different from the olden days of hospital indifference toward the patients' desires. What a wonderful way to change their inhumane reputation.

After you have gained permission for husbands to be present with their wives in the delivery room of your local hospital, the next step is to let them bring their cameras. Let us supply you with some ammunition to convince your doctor and the hospital administrator that pictures are a good thing. The reasons are medical, physical, and spiritual.

DADDY PICTURES

1. "Daddy pictures" are of benefit to the husband-wife relationship. They are objective proof of true togetherness in parenthood. Birth is thereby illustrated as a shared experience.

   Such pictures place the moment of birth on a similar level of familial importance with the marriage ceremony, wedding anniversaries, and annual anniversaries of this moment known as "birthdays." Aren't these all occasions to be preserved by picture taking? Why take birthday pictures on subsequent anniversaries but ignore the original and main event?

   These pictures bind the marriage bonds tighter and make family life richer, more meaningful. In my observation the divorce rate is significantly low in couples who tenderly preserve via pictures the memory of the moment of the birth of their children.

2. The role of photographer adds purpose to the role of the husband. In family-centered childbirth the low incidence of postpartum psychoses (nervous breakdowns) of mothers is related to the useful rather than useless part played by the husband. Women can subconsciously resent absent, passive husbands who take no active interest in the birth of their children. Dr. Carl L. Kline, in a medical article (*American Journal of Obstetrics & Gynecology,* volume 69, 1955, pp. 748–757) discussing the cause of postpartum psychoses, states, "One of the most frequently expressed sources of resentment of a wife toward her husband is passivity on the part of the husband."

    "Daddy pictures" are vivid proof of the husband's presence and his active interest. Many women have remarked how their husband's whole attitude toward being a father improved and in some instances changed completely after he was taught the importance of his active role in childbirth.

3. These pictures may be beneficial in the psychological and spiritual development of the child, as suggested in the first part of this chapter.

4. The pictures are valuable in prenatal education. They give reassurance to the inexperienced. Probably no aspect of prenatal preparation is as effective in dispelling fear and anxiety in the inexperienced couple as for them to study copies of pictures taken by other parents.

It appears obvious that our main reason for inviting the husband to share in the birth experience is simply that his wife will be so radiantly happy in her achievement that he shouldn't be left out.

And there is really no good reason why, if they wish, husbands shouldn't be allowed cameras. Don't abuse the privilege and come dragging along enormous amounts of photographic equipment, but use just a simple camera you hold in your hand.

No ill effect possibly attributable to these "daddy pictures" has ever occurred. "Infection—cameras are dirty," some opponents may claim. Yet our hospital has not had any higher infection rate. "The photographer will interfere with the function of the nurses." Give him permission and directions where to stand to take pictures. All of this is dramatized and clearly outlined to the husband at the prenatal class on labor and birth.

A few progressive hospitals allow siblings and even friends of the patient in the birth rooms or borning rooms today. An excellent book to prepare the brothers and sisters of the baby is *Children at Birth* (Academy Publications, 2008), written and worked up by the entire Hathaway family and available at www.bradleybirth.com. It won't take much explaining to tell these children where babies come from.

If a few "medical Daniels" hadn't dared to be different, we would still be treating all diseases with leeches and bloodletting. Yet it takes courage indeed to stand with a new minority against an established majority. Permission for husbands, siblings, friends, or cameras in delivery rooms cannot be based upon a majority vote of the medical staff; the concepts are too new.

The administrator has to follow his own convictions. Your doctor similarly will run up against a lot of doctor opposition. Some of this will be good-natured kidding, some will be vicious. He will need a deep conviction in his innermost soul that husband-shared unanesthetized childbirth is the better way, and he will need intestinal fortitude to persevere toward this goal against the many obstacles placed in his path. Is it worth all the trouble? Ask the parents who have experienced it, ask them!

I retired from obstetrical practice without a single maternal mortality. I am deeply and sincerely convinced that the constant presence of a loved and loving husband serves to foster a state of serenity in the mother's mind that is comparable to or a part of the religious serenity that has aided some mothers for centuries to follow their instinctive abilities calmly and give birth actively to their babies. Your presence as a trained and loving helper will foster that serenity in your wife as she becomes a mother.

18

NUTRITION IN PREGNANCY

From the Work of Dr. Tom Brewer

In the video "Nutrition in Pregnancy" (Academy Communications), Dr. Bradley introduced Dr. Brewer by saying, "There is a pioneer in the field of nutrition in pregnancy, Dr. Thomas Brewer, and he has worked very hard to stress to people the importance of maintaining good protein input in pregnancy, and his many writings and extensive work—and research he has done, including his book on the *Metabolic Toxemia of Late Pregnancy*—make him an authority in the field."

What a mother eats can make a difference in her health, and the health of her unborn child.

It is shocking to realize that the United States' infant mortality rate is twenty-sixth compared to other countries, according to *Pediatrics* (volume 119, number 2, February 2007). This means that countries, including Sweden, Switzerland, Canada, Germany, the United Kingdom, Australia, Japan, even Cuba and Hong Kong, have lower infant mortality rates than the U.S.

If we were talking about sports or the Olympics this would be a national disaster. The problem is that infant or maternal death isn't a major news event. People don't want to talk about it. Occasionally you see or hear stories about the high cost of low birth-weight babies in neonatal intensive care units. This can lead to a high ongoing cost, including medical and education expenses. The same journal article showed the incidence of babies weighing less than five and a half pounds (twenty-five hundred grams) has gone up to 8.2 percent and is climbing, especially with so many inductions and cesareans.

Dr. Brewer began working as a junior medical student at Charity Hospital, in New Orleans. He saw lots of women with toxemia of pregnancy, some with convulsions, in comas, and even some who died.

He started asking patients what they ate. What they liked to eat. He took total health histories and found that women who ate well, did well.

Further he found that a well-balanced high-protein (eighty to one hundred grams a day) diet was essential for making, as he proudly referred to them, "Blue Ribbon Babies." Babies whose moms were on this well-balanced diet tended to be healthier and the moms did not have toxemia, which he attributed directly to this diet.

Dr. Brewer spent eleven years studying diet and outcomes in a nutritional program in Contra Costa County, California. He worked with low-income women and virtually eliminated toxemia, low birth weight, and prematurity.

Today there are a number of labels for the disease that historically was called toxemia including: preeclampsia, eclampsia (seizures), PIH (pregnancy-induced hypertension), HELLP syndrome (H-hemolysis, EL-elevated liver enzymes, LP-low platelet count).

With a lot of help from mothers who wanted healthy babies and information from the United States Department of Agriculture, Dr. Brewer came up with a basic, inexpensive diet women could follow to increase the chance of having a healthy baby.

THE BASICS ARE:

Every day of the week you and your baby should have:

1. One quart (four glasses) or more of milk
2. Two eggs
3. Two servings of protein
4. Two good servings of fresh green leafy vegetables
5. Four or more slices (or servings) of whole grains
6. One citrus fruit
7. Three pats of butter (fats or oils)
8. Other fruits and vegetables

Also include in your diet:

1. A serving of whole-grain cereal such as oatmeal or granola
2. A yellow- or orange-colored fruit or vegetable (five times a week)
3. Liver once a week (if you like it)
4. Whole baked potato (three times a week)
5. Plenty of fluids, water, juice, etc.
6. Salt food to taste, for a safe increase in blood volume

MILK

Milk provides protein, calcium, fats, and other essential vitamins and minerals. These are important for bones, muscle growth, muscle contraction, and nerve transmission. They are also essential for healthy blood, they ease insomnia, and help regulate the heartbeat. Dietary fats in regular milk are important for the development of the fetus as well as young children.

Recommendation: Four or more servings per day

Note: If you are allergic to any food, discuss alternatives with your health-care provider and with your instructor.

SUBSTITUTES FOR MILK

Dr. Brewer has shown pregnant women that a well-balanced diet, that includes milk, can help them have a healthier pregnancy and healthier babies. Adequate protein and calcium have even been associated with a decrease in serious complications of pregnancy called preeclampsia, HELLP syndrome, or toxemia.

Milk contains many important elements in a well-balanced diet including calcium, protein, folic acid, zinc, vitamin A, vitamin B_{12}, vitamin D, potassium, phosphorus, niacin, riboflavin, and many more. It is possible to substitute for milk. Some people are allergic, vegetarian, or prefer to get their calcium, protein, calories, and other elements from other foods. Some people who are allergic to milk find they have no problems with other dairy products such as cottage cheese or yogurt. Milk is an easy to obtain, inexpensive source of protein, calcium, and calories. If you choose to substitute, do it carefully! Each person must decide what is right for them.

Recommendation: Four or more servings per day

Note: If you are allergic to any food, discuss alternatives with your health-care provider and with your instructor.

EGGS

Eggs provide protein, vitamins, and minerals, including vitamin A, the anti-infection vitamin. Added together, milk and eggs provide a protein, vitamin, mineral, and calorie foundation for the rest of the diet, and provide the additional cholesterol necessary during pregnancy, which is essential for fetal brain development.

Recommendation: Two per day

Note: If you are allergic to any food, discuss alternatives with your health-care provider and with your instructor.

PROTEIN

Protein provides amino acids, which are the building blocks of the body. Important for healthy bones, teeth, muscles, brain—everything! Inadequate protein intake can lead to fatigue, cravings for sweets, a lack of appetite, toxemia, swelling, and premature labor.

ADDING PROTEIN TO YOUR DIET

Dairy foods and eggs are a great complete source of protein and are relatively inexpensive. They can be added to lots of recipes that will boost your protein intake. Add to sauces, cakes, breads, pasta, salads, drinks without basically changing what you first set out to make.

SUBSTITUTIONS

You may substitute proteins if you wish, being sure your proteins are complete, and that you get approximately eighty to one hundred grams per day. If you substitute, also be sure all the elements necessary for a well-balanced diet are eaten every day.

Recommendation: Two servings per day

Note: If you are allergic to any food, discuss alternatives with your health-care provider and with your instructor.

GREENS

Fresh, dark green vegetables are rich in vitamins (particularly A and B complex) and minerals, which are necessary to help your body use the protein in other foods. These are also high in folic acid, which is essential for good growth, and which protects against neurological disorders and spina bifida. Greens also play a role in the formation of red blood cells. A deficiency could lead to anemia. The darker the greens, the higher the concentration of vitamins and minerals.

Recommendation: Two servings per day

Note: If you are allergic to any food, discuss alternatives with your health-care provider and with your instructor.

WHOLE GRAINS

These are excellent sources of carbohydrates you need to fuel your body. If you have too few carbohydrates, your body burns the protein you eat for energy, thus robbing you and your baby of the building blocks for tissue growth and repair. Carbohydrates from whole grains also are a good source of B vitamins, which are necessary for growth and the normal functioning of nerve tissue and energy.

Recommendation: Four or more servings per day

Note: If you are allergic to any food, discuss alternatives with your health-care provider and with your instructor.

CITRUS FOODS HIGH IN VITAMIN C

Vitamin C is important for the body's ability to manufacture collagen, the substance that holds tissue together. Without adequate C, your uterus is not going to be as strong and may not perform as well in labor. Vitamin C is crucial in the body's defense system against infection and in improving iron absorption.

Recommendation: One or more servings per day

Note: If you are allergic to any food, discuss alternatives with your health-care provider and with your instructor.

BUTTER (FATS AND OILS)

Fats and oils are needed in your diet to help your body absorb the fat-soluble vitamins A, D, E, and K. Fats and oils also contribute to a fine-textured (stretchable) skin. They are concentrated sources of calories. The food energy or calorie need is increased in pregnancy to a minimum of 2500–3000 calories per day.

Recommendation: Three or more servings per day

Note: If you are allergic to any food, discuss alternatives with your health-care provider and with your instructor.

YELLOW AND ORANGE FRUITS AND VEGETABLES

These foods are high in vitamin A, which is known for its role in preventing infection. During pregnancy, when the pressure of the growing uterus on the bladder is constant, extra vitamin A helps protect you against bladder and kidney infection and is also good for the skin.

Recommendation: Five times a week

Note: If you are allergic to any food, discuss alternatives with your health-care provider and with your instructor.

SALT

Salt is an essential nutrient. If you were to completely eliminate salt from your diet, your body would cease to function. There is an increased need for salt during pregnancy because of the extra demands the baby places on the mother's body.

Use common sense; let your body tell you how much salt you need.

You will know that your body needs more salt when your food tastes flat. Women who have conditioned themselves not to eat salt must be especially careful and may have to look for the symptoms of salt deficiency in addition to paying attention to their taste buds.

The salt that you shake on your food is just one source for the sodium you need. There is also a good amount in most high-protein foods, such as milk, meats, and seafood, and in some vegetables. Kelp powder and soy sauce are also good sources of sodium.

You need extra salt if you live in a hot climate, do vigorous exercise, or sweat (perspire) a lot.

Salt can help with swelling and leg cramps. Without enough salt (hyponatremia), you are more likely to develop either of these. It helps to maintain an adequate blood volume for safety.

WATER (FLUIDS)

Water is essential for good health. Pure water (nothing mixed in) is best for rehydration of the body. Bottled or filtered water may be necessary, depending on your water source at home. Water accounts for 75 percent of your baby's total body weight at birth. It acts as a solvent and catalyst for biological reactions. Lack of water leads to dehydration, which can lead to over a 20 percent reduction of energy output. Dehydration can also lead to headaches during pregnancy. Water deficiency can lead to declined circulation (low blood flow), hypovolemia (low blood volume), oligohydramnios (low amniotic fluid volume), which can trigger premature labor.

Note: Water without adequate salt intake leads to an imbalance, making it hard for your body to absorb and retain fluids.

Recommendation: DRINK TO THIRST—OFTEN!!!
(According to your environment and energy output.)

Be careful about your source of water.

Be careful of some bottled water. Read the labels. Some of them have additives such as magnesium sulfate ($MgSO_4$), which is a laxative (muscle relaxant), and is used to stop labors. This is commonly known as Epsom salts.

If you are a vegetarian or a vegan, read *Pregnancy, Childbirth, and the Vegan Diet* by Dr. Michael Klaper.

THE BEST NUTRITION FOR YOUR BABY IS BREAST MILK

SOME OF THE ADVANTAGES OF BREAST-FEEDING

1. Breast milk is the perfect food for your baby—even formula companies, the American Academy of Pediatrics, and the United States government agree on this!
2. Breast-feeding is best for the mother's health after birth.
3. Breast milk is the only thing your baby needs for at least the first six to nine months.
4. Breast milk is a live fluid—digests easily and rapidly.
5. Breast milk is not as likely to constipate the baby as formula.
6. Breast-fed babies smell much, much better!
7. Breast-fed babes have less likelihood of:
   Serious digestive upsets
   Diaper rash
   Respiratory infections, etc.
8. Breast-fed babies are much easier to travel with.
9. Breast-feeding causes secretion of prolactin (mothering hormone).
10. Breast-fed babies are easier to feed at night, you and Mom get more sleep.
11. Breast milk is readily available, properly mixed and heated.
12. Breast-feeding lowers the risk of breast cancer.

NUTRITION PLAYS A ROLE IN CESAREAN SURGERY

A mother who has been well nourished during pregnancy:
. . . has a better chance of having a uterus that is strong and efficient so cesarean surgery is less likely to be necessary.

. . . has less chance of postpartum infection, whether she has a natural birth or a cesarean surgery. Will heal better and faster.

. . . if she has a cesarean surgery has a better chance for a VBAC (vaginal birth after cesarean) next time.

Nutrition is the foundation of a healthy pregnancy. Making sure you have a complete diet, including proteins, vegetables, fruits, starches, grains, water, salt, and fluids, etc., will give you the building blocks necessary for your body to help create an exceptional new person, your baby!

Your body needs to have the essential elements readily available when needed, to construct this new life inside you. For instance, if a car were being manufactured and one or more elements were not available then the car would be deficient and would not meet your high expectations. So having whatever the body needs in your system can help give your baby the best start possible.

19

PREGNANCY PROBLEMS: NATURAL PREVENTION

The best way to treat a disease or problem is not to have it. Preventive medicine is just now coming into its own as a division of the healing arts. This so-called holistic medicine treats the human being not as a robot or machine but as a total being made in the image of God, with complex interacting of body-mind-soul relationships.

Natural childbirth is truly a facet of holistic medicine and I consider it to be probably the most important aspect. Here we are dealing with creation itself. The future of the human race will be determined by the elimination of drugs and chemicals in mothers' and fathers' bodies, to produce intelligent babies whose brains are clear. These children will almost certainly grow into their maximum potential as intelligent adults capable of solving our many problems.

NUTRITION

To ward off the need for drugs, prevention of obstetrical complications is indicated. Nutrition leads the list in importance. A proper high-protein, balanced diet helps prevent toxemia of late pregnancy, reduces the risk of premature labor, makes the cervix more flexible for dilatation in labor, builds body resistance to give natural immunity against infections, and provides proper requirements for growth of the developing baby. Read *Metabolic Toxemia of Late Pregnancy,* by Tom Brewer, M.D. (Academy Publications, 2005).

EMOTIONAL STABILITY

Emotional stability from self-confidence, acquired through awareness of what is required in the role of mother, changes a "worrywart" into a poised obstetrical athlete whose serene mind will prevent her baby's being "uptight." She will accept the little pressure pains of an enlarging uterus without complaint or panic. Emotional disharmony and chronic tension are harmful to the body, making it prone to ulcers, spastic colon, premature labor, and increased susceptibility to infections of all kinds. An interested, involved, understanding husband who is himself emotionally stable helps immeasurably.

SPIRITUAL

I am convinced that spiritual attunement is also part of the picture, being true to your own beliefs seems to be important; for I have observed that those individuals with deep, abiding faith in God, those who have that inner peace, which passeth all understanding, are less prone to colds, infections of all kinds, and, of course, the many ailments of inner spasticity. Blessed is the baby born unto a couple who have this awareness. Babies are truly blessings from God; if you don't believe this, ask the couple who want one and for some reason can't have it.

Let's itemize some of the physical problems of pregnancy, to see if we can't in some way prevent them. Natural ways of treating them, if they occur, will follow, but prevention takes precedence.

THE COMMON COLD

Some people nearly always have a cold; others hardly ever do. What is the difference between them? We don't really know the last word on bodily immunity. Emotional and spiritual disharmony undoubtedly plays a role, as does contact with other people. The hermit who lives in isolation seldom gets a cold. The office worker bottled up with many other people gets far more exposure.

We can't all be hermits, but during the cold seasons (spring and fall) and during known epidemics, stay away as much as possible from crowds of people. Send your husband to the grocery store; his body is not growing the baby and so is more immune and resistant.

DO NOT OVERTIRE

Do not overtire yourself when pregnant. Get that extra hour of sleep, and whatever you're doing, stop and rest when you get tired. Take your prenatal vitamin supplements dutifully and nibble on fresh fruit between meals regularly. I'm convinced extra vitamin C via fresh fruits helps ward off colds.

MOISTURIZER OR HUMIDIFIER

If you live in a dry climate, have a moisturizer in your bedroom or a humidifier on the furnace. Do not blow your nose violently. Fragile mucosa and blood vessels will break, affording doorways for viruses. Using your little finger, keep your nostrils lubricated with your favorite moisturizer to prevent cracks.

WILL YOURSELF . . .

Last, but not least, will yourself not to get a cold. As you go to sleep at bedtime, direct your subconscious mind to resist colds. There is an altered state of consciousness as you enter the sleep state which exposes the more suggestible subconscious mind, which is truly in charge of your body. Give it a try.

BLADDER INFECTIONS

Women are more prone to bladder infections than men. This is due to many factors, but the first is that women just don't drink enough water, for two reasons. First, drinking water may make you need to go to the bathroom more often and perspire more, and some people think that's not ladylike! Second, women can get so busy they have to put off going to the bathroom. Job pressures cause many women to avoid drinking enough water. Some examples are bank tellers who may be too busy to leave their station, executives in long meetings, or women who need to spend time anywhere bathrooms are scarce. Some women train themselves to go to the bathroom at home only because of concerns over cleanliness.

PERSPIRATION

Now, perspiration may not be ladylike, but it is definitely mother-like. Not only is the pregnant woman urinating for two people, which requires extra water, but the circulation of an increased volume of blood increases fluid loss from the skin, mostly insensible and invisible fluid loss from evaporation as well as occasional beads of sweat. Therefore, extra water is needed; eight to ten glasses each day.

"GOTTA GO" FEELING . . . NEED MORE WATER

Strong, concentrated urine from inadequate fluid intake irritates the bladder mucosa and makes it more prone to infection as well as producing an urgency to urinate, a "gotta go" feeling when the bladder isn't really full.

It is hard to convince mothers that drinking extra water dilutes the urine so that it is not irritating to the bladder, with consequent decreased frequency of urination.

A physical factor that makes women more prone to bladder infections is the relative shortness of the urethra, the tube that drains the urine to the outside. Having less space to travel, bacteria concentrate in a small area.

"DON'TS"

Because of the shortness of this tube we suggest a series of "don'ts" to prevent bladder infections: Don't cross your legs. Little girls, feeling the urgent need to empty their bladder as urine descends into the upper portion of the urethra, find that by crossing their legs they can squeeze the urine back up into the bladder; this fools them into thinking they don't really have to urinate and can continue to play. Women know better than this, but society dictates they should cross their legs to be "ladylike." Regardless of the reason, the effect is the same. Bacteria are squeezed into and up the urethra, to cause infection. Mothers, as was stressed in the chapter on coaches' training rules, should sit with their legs apart, preferably on the floor, tailor-fashion.

PANTIES

Don't wear panties. Cloth between the legs, whatever the material, mixes skin bacteria and bacteria from the adjacent rectal opening, innoculating the urinary opening with multiple bacteria. A bare bottom is a healthy bottom, and a long, floppy skirt worn around the house without underwear is appropriate to this problem.

I strongly feel that the current rash of vaginal infections is related to women dressing in men's-style clothing. I'm an old square who thinks women look graceful and feminine in long skirts with lace and frills to accentuate their femininity. Pioneer women wore long skirts with no underclothes—at least for working—and had far fewer bladder infections than modern women who wear slacks, especially tight, rigid denims, and panty hose. In addition, the exercises of squatting and tailor sitting can be performed so much more easily in a large, loose skirt than in tight-fitting slacks. Don't just act like a lady; dress like one.

DON'T OVER BATHE

Don't over bathe your vaginal area. This is the most over bathed area of a woman's body, because of the excretory openings, I suppose. Vigorous scrubbing with lavish amounts of soap dries out protective natural skin oils and causes breaks and cracks in the skin of the urethral opening as well as the thin, sensitive lips of the vagina. As stressed before, it doesn't matter how mild the TV ads claim soap to be, or how much moisturizer has been added; soap is soap. It is designed to remove grease and oil from the skin, but it also removes natural skin oil, leaving parched, dry skin. Warm bathwater with unperfumed bath oil in it will readily dissolve perspiration and bodily secretions, so soap is not really necessary.

HAND CREAM

As the hands are used more and get dirty more than any other part of the body, they are washed more often with soap and get chapped. To counteract this soap effect, hand cream was invented to at least partially replace depleted skin oil. Women are noted for applying cream and oils to their hands and face. At the risk of being labeled a male chauvinist, I believe they are ignoring an important part of their anatomy. I recommend that a good hand cream, preferably non-perfumed, be used daily after bathing on the lips of the vagina and the adjacent skin of the legs and perineum, where skin rubs against skin to produce friction.

SKIN FLEXIBLE

Keeping this skin flexible so it will stretch better when the baby is born has been stressed before, but the application of moisturizer also prevents the cracking of the skin that allows bacteria to enter and start infections. Intact, healthy skin is a marvelous natural protective barrier to infection. One can roll an apple around in dirt and it will not become infected or get rotten unless there is a break in the apple skin. Even the tiniest opening will allow bacteria to enter.

LOVEMAKING

Don't make love on your back. The rather quaint and unnatural position of American lovemaking in which the woman lies on her back and her big, heavy husband lies on top of her is often referred to as the "missionary position." This label supposedly comes from the reactions of natives in a distant land, who, peeking into the missionaries' tent to see how they made love, were amazed at their odd position. As previously stressed, the man shouldn't be on top, as the weight of his body compresses the baby against his wife's back, which can be harmful as well as uncomfortable. With the wife on top or by his side, she can back away or give a bit if the pressure is excessive. Also, she can angle her hips and legs so that the angle of insertion of the thrusting penis does not put excessive pressure on the urethra, in the front of the vagina.

KEGEL

Don't forget to do your Kegel exercises. If you don't empty your bladder completely, bacteria will grow in the stale urine that remains and will start bladder infections. Having a good strong Kegel muscle and knowing how to use it makes for more efficient emptying of the bladder.

VAGINAL INFECTIONS

Practically the same preventive measures apply here as with bladder infections, for the bladder and vagina are next-door neighbors. Because light hardly ever shines on the opening of the vagina—unless you're a regularly practicing nudist (and they do have far fewer vaginal infections)—the vagina with its constant moisture is an ideal medium for the growth of molds and fungi.

DOUCHES

Nature in her wisdom creates an acid-producing bacteria that exists in the healthy vagina and helps prevent the growth of invading bacteria and molds. Our main caution here is: don't take douches and wash out nature's protective mucus.

UNDERWEAR

Also, the irritation of perspiration and mucus-retaining underwear produces infection. In men, it is known as "jock itch," as tight-fitting jockey shorts or jockstraps retain perspiration and irritate and infect adjacent skin. In babies, we call the same thing "diaper rash"; in women, I call it "panty rash." To protect your baby, take off the diaper and place it on the crib mattress. Similarly, if you want to prevent panty rash, take off the offending garment.

I cringe at miniskirts, not just because I think long skirts are more feminine and graceful, but because with miniskirts, not wearing panties becomes a social problem. But even if you must wear short skirts for the sake of fashion, I suggest wearing a comfortable big wrap-type skirt or a caftan at home.

WET BATHING SUIT

If you live in a warm climate and, following our advice, swim for exercise, do not sit around the pool for long periods of time in a wet bathing suit, or vaginal infections may result.

FLU

Both stomach and intestinal flu are caused by viruses. The only preventive measures are those listed for the common cold. During flu epidemics, play hermit and stay away from crowds. Get adequate rest, take your vitamins, eat a proper diet, and use a positive attitude to build up a natural immunity.

BRUISES, LACERATIONS, AND PUNCTURE WOUNDS

Being pregnant, you bruise more easily. Blood vessels carrying one-third more blood break more easily. Bodily energies going to grow a baby are depleted elsewhere, so do not indulge in contact sports, wear shoes when roughing it, and be careful of falling—your balance is goofy.

POSTPARTUM INFECTIONS

Natural childbirth itself, with a minimum of vaginal examinations, a reduced need for forceps, awareness of the dangers of internal electronic fetal monitors, which pierce the baby's protective layer (its skin), the spontaneous, unassisted separation and passage of the placenta, immediate breast-feeding to properly contract the uterus—all these help prevent the dreaded "childbed fever."

Today with some doctors using more and more interventions, they find themselves needing to use antibiotic drugs hoping to cure infections. This is often done in advance, just in case. It used to be thought infections were caused only by unsterile procedures, now we know that both healthy and sometimes harmful microorganisms live and thrive inside the vagina and may be forced up into the uterus by exams or by devices, especially after the bag of waters has broken. These can be the cause of life-threatening diseases and infections. There is no such thing as a "sterile" vaginal exam.

THE BREAST

Nurse for five to ten minutes on one breast, then as long as the baby wants on the other side. The baby often goes to sleep on the second side. If baby still wants to nurse, start over again. Newborns may nurse as often as every twenty minutes to three hours; each baby has its own pattern. Alternating back and forth helps keep a uniform pull on each breast, which helps prevent plugged milk ducts and breast infections. Frequent nursing will help establish a good milk supply. Check with La Leche League and *The Bradley Method Student Workbook* about positioning the baby at the breast to prevent sore, cracked nipples.

Let the baby alternate which breast is used first and mark your bra with a safety pin, so you don't have to rely on memory, at least at first. Later on, you can tell by feel which one is fuller.

FEVER

Do not try to prevent fever; some degree of hyperthermia is the body's way of treating infection. Some women notice an increased body temperature when their milk comes in. This is generally normal. A temperature over 101 degrees by mouth should be discussed with your health team.

HEMORRHOIDS

These tender, often painful bumps in or around the rectal opening are actually varicose veins of the rectum. Like varicose veins anywhere, they become hot and exceedingly sore if the blood in them stagnates enough to form a clot, or thrombus. The best treatment is prevention, by proper eating and fluid intake so that the bowel contents are not hard or constipated. Also effective is performing the natural-childbirth exercises that lift the heavy uterus and its contents off the rectum. Pelvic rocking and Kegels are especially helpful. We jokingly state that the best preventive measure is to pick your parents carefully, for these weak rectal veins are inherited.

VARICOSE VEINS OF THE LEGS

Thanks to the natural-childbirth exercises, proper social exercises, and the wearing of nonrestrictive clothing (girdles and tight elastic garters have to go!), we hardly ever see these problems anymore. In spite of inherited weakness of veins, circulation can be maintained by following our unladylike but mother-like exercises around the home, supplemented by swimming, bicycle riding, etc., once a week throughout pregnancy. These things do make a difference.

GENITAL HERPES INFECTION

Genital herpes or herpes simplex II is a sexually transmitted disease that undoubtedly spreads into and from small breaks in the delicate skin of the vaginal lips. Herpes simplex I, a relative of genital herpetic infection, makes so-called fever blisters on the oral lips. Good skiers know enough to put heavy lip balm on their oral lips to prevent the wind and the sun from forming chapped, cracked lips that allow herpetic invasion. Good natural-childbirth mothers, even when not pregnant, know enough to routinely avoid the drying-out action of soap on the vaginal lips and use thick hand cream daily to prevent chapping and cracking.

I saw very few cases of pelvic herpes, especially in women who were following our principles. The legs-apart tailor-sitting position with a full skirt and no underwear undoubtedly plays an important role in prevention of this dreadful, untreatable (at this time) infection.

Today, there seems to be an increase of cases of herpes. In the book *The Birth Center* (Prentice Hall, 1986), Victor Berman, M.D., and Salee Berman, C.N.M., discuss herpes: herpes simplex type II, or genital herpes, is a virus that poses a threat to the baby. Transplacental infection (i.e., infection through the bloodstream to the baby) is possible but rare.

Current medical opinion holds that the baby usually becomes infected by direct contact with the infected area during vaginal birth. The virus attacks the immature nervous system of the newborn infant and can produce devastating effects that may lead to brain damage and death. In the past, if the mother has had an active herpes simplex type II lesion within three weeks of going into labor, the general practice has been to perform a cesarean birth to protect the baby. However, if repeated cervical cultures are negative, it is now considered safe to have a normal vaginal birth.

The Bermans also recommend the following vitamin therapy as a preventive measure: vitamin C, L-lysine, and zinc tend to decrease the frequency and severity of herpes symptoms. The recommended maintenance dosages are:

2,000 milligrams of vitamin C
600 milligrams of L-lysine
50 milligrams of zinc

These amounts should be taken daily and during an active outbreak should be doubled. Vitamin C is a water-soluble vitamin, L-lysine is an amino acid. Zinc is a nontoxic mineral routinely required by the body. As with any supplementation take care to watch for allergic reactions. Always check with a health-care provider who is knowledgeable in this area before starting treatment.

CONSTIPATION

The era of the glorification of bowel movements has long since passed. When I was a child, my dutiful mother "cleaned me out" every Saturday night with castor oil in preparation for going to church Sunday morning. I violently protested that my bowel contents couldn't be "dirty," as I hadn't eaten any dirt, and why should the residue from digesting what I had eaten be "dirty"? All to no avail. There is no more addictive drug than laxatives. The poor bowel quits doing its work unless stimulated by drugs, and the dosage has to be steadily increased over the years to get the resistant bowel to work.

Sometimes prospective mothers get so busy that they ignore the urge to move their bowels, putting it off until a more convenient time. The bowel does not like to be ignored. After a few times it refuses to give the message anymore. If this has happened, try to reestablish the gastrocolic reflex. This is a message customarily sent by the stomach to the colon in the mornings when breakfast is imminent. Just the fragrance of cooking will sometimes do it. The three meals eaten during the day are digested during the night, so that the residue fills the colon as you sleep.

The urge to move the bowels is telegraphed as a nerve reflex telling the bowel: "Empty out, more is coming." The result is "regularity," or bowel movements in the morning. If you have destroyed this reflex by ignoring it, then try reestablishing it by regularly trying to move the bowels after breakfast.

Do not depend upon harsh chemicals or bowel stimulants. Anyone who follows the dietary advice in this book should never need chemical bowel softeners. The high-protein, high-roughage diet and adequate fluids automatically produce soft bowel movements, so drugs are not usually necessary.

20

PREGNANCY PROBLEMS: NATURAL HEALING

The human body you were given is itself a marvelous mechanism for healing. There is always a "doctor in the house" for self-healing.

"GRANDMOTHER TREATMENT"

Before you reach into the drug cabinet or present yourself to a doctor of medicine for a prescription, give your body a chance first. If what I respectfully refer to as "grandmother treatment" doesn't work, then go see your doctor for help. Grandmother treatment is accomplished by imagining that you are a pioneer, living in the wilderness. There is no drugstore or doctor available, and you have to treat yourself without drugs. Cooperate with nature; don't subdue it with drugs.

DRUGS IN PREGNANCY . . .
HARMFUL TO FETUS

As far as I'm concerned, all drugs taken in pregnancy are potentially or actually harmful to the fetus. Take them as a last resort only, as properly prescribed by a drug-aware physician.

As a father, this approach won't hurt you one bit, either, for avoidance of drugs is good for your body, too. Modern geneticists feel that if men cleared their bodies of chemicals and drugs before getting their wives pregnant, there would be fewer defective babies.

We are here prescribing the horse sense of grandmother treatment to otherwise healthy young people, not to the chronically ill, the debilitated, or the elderly.

COMMON COLD

I am vehemently against the idle use of chemicals to help the ordinary symptoms or nuisances of infections to go away. I protest that some symptoms are purposeful and represent part of nature's way of helping the body heal the infection.

Let me illustrate by an example—the use of vasoconstrictive nasal sprays to help keep your virus-infected stuffed-up nose open. I stoutly maintain it is stopped up for a reason, to avoid being used when it is infected and sore. If your thumb is infected and sore, it will get well faster if you don't use it for a while. Likewise your nose. "But I can't breathe!" you protest. Sure you can; just use your mouth. "But it gets so dry." So chew crushed ice, make some Popsicles in the freezer from fresh lemon, lime, or orange juice, or concentrated apple juice, with honey as a sweetener. This not only tastes good but moistens your mouth, elevates your blood sugar, provides extra vitamin C, etc.

Rest.   If your body must muster its defenses to attack the invader, for heaven's sake rest until you get well and give your body all its energy for the task at hand. The wise grandmother would agree.

Promote perspiration.   In horses and men, says my wife, we refer to it as "sweat." In ladies it is called "perspiration." By any name, promote it. Grandmother precedes the bed rest with a good long warm bath, followed by plenty of covers on the bed or hot-water bottles or, in my ancient day, hot soapstones. When you get sweaty, don't immediately uncover to cool off, but keep sweating; it's good for you. I know sweating is not socially acceptable in the drawing room, but it is essential to health in the bedroom when you have a cold.

Force oral fluids.   In order to sweat, you have to have something to sweat with—a fundamental law. Just before going to bed, try a cup of the juice of a whole lemon and a tablespoon of honey, with boiling water to fill the teacup—then stay covered and perspire. Hot chicken soup is an excellent source of protein, and the soup fumes also loosen phlegm and clear the sinuses— smart grandmothers. Any very hot liquid of your choice is beneficial from the heat standpoint alone.

Gargle with hot salt water.   This is particularly appropriate upon arising and before breakfast, as phlegm and mucus accumulate in the posterior nasal and sinus areas during sleep as the result of a horizontal position. These substances need to be eliminated by gargling just before eating, or intestinal upset can follow from the drainage accompanying food to the stomach.

Humidify the bedroom air.   Moisture particles known as "dew" that occur in the air at night are carriers of pollen, dust, and other irritants to the already irritated upper respiratory tract. Keep them out by closing the windows and increasing the moisture in the bedroom so that it is more concentrated than the outside air. In summertime, a cold-air humidifier is indicated, in wintertime, a steam vaporizer. No chemicals or drugs should be added; just water vapor is all that is needed. This also promotes perspiration and reduces the need for coughing in order to clear irritants.

COUGHING

Don't fight coughs with chemical suppressants. Coughs serve a purpose in the common cold by keeping infected mucus from descending into the trachea and lungs, thus creating a lower respiratory tract infection out of the upper one. Now, of course, with pneumonia, bronchitis, or other severe infections, your doctor will have to use drugs, but not for a common cold.

EAR INFECTIONS

This complication in upper respiratory infections should be treated promptly by your physician. No grandmother treatment is effective. I'm convinced it occurs less when people refrain from blowing their nose.

LARYNGITIS

If the larynx, or voice box, becomes infected with a virus, the basic treatment applies, with the addition of one admonition: shut up! Don't talk; give your voice box a rest until it heals.

BLADDER INFECTIONS

The best treatment, of course, is prevention (see previous chapter), but if in spite of precautions you get the typical urgency, frequency, and painful urination, again, do simple things first. Force oral fluids, including water, soups, gelatin, fruit juices, etc. Drinking cranberry juice or eating cranberries causes an acidity in the urine that may suppress bacterial infection. As with all infections, get extra bed rest; be a lazybones. Also take a long leisurely warm sitz bath. Sit in warm water while reading something to keep you from being bored. Long baths are best.

SOAP AND BATH OILS

Keep soap and bath oils off the urethra, or bladder opening; they tend to irritate. The purpose of the warm sitz baths is not cleanliness but application of heat.

If the symptoms don't clear up in a day or two, consult your medical team.

VAGINAL INFECTIONS

Here again, the best treatment is prevention. No grandmother treatment is as effective as a doctor's diagnosing the cause and treating the infection with local chemicals. I do not believe the vaginal mucosa absorbs enough of the chemical to harm the baby.

FLU

This is a virus for which no alleviating drug or chemical has yet been found. When the virus "bug" affects your throat and upper respiratory tract, the previously described treatment for the common cold applies.

It can also attack your stomach or upper alimentary canal, with resultant severe nausea and eventual vomiting. Do not take drugs to try to stop the vomiting. Treat your stomach gently for a while by giving it easy-to-digest foods only, for a day or two. The best liquid to start with is freshly squeezed orange juice in shaved ice, then drink ice-cold lemon-flavored carbonated soda—only minimal amounts at first. Slowly add light soups, gelatin, and other liquids. Soon, solids may be resumed, but avoid highly spiced or hard-to-digest foods for a while. Contact your medical team if vomiting persists, or you become dehydrated.

DIARRHEA

Should the virus attack the lower alimentary canal and rather violent diarrhea and cramps occur, use the sensible heat treatment of warm baths and extra bed rest to restore your body's reserves for overcoming the infection.

I'm against chemicals to try to stop diarrhea. Nature has a reason for everything, I maintain, and you will overcome the infection sooner if you let nature take its course. Making jellylike bowel movements by taking various forms of pectin is totally illogical. You're treating your mind and handicapping your bowel.

Similarly, chemicals that prevent the cramps of a hyperactive bowel by paralyzing it, so it can't clear itself out, are equally illogical and interfere with healing. Give nature a chance first. Of course, long-persisting diarrhea should be investigated by your doctor, but you will be amazed at how quickly your body can handle a flu virus if you just give it a chance and don't interfere.

LACERATIONS AND PUNCTURE WOUNDS

Long, deep cuts may require the attention of a doctor, who can determine the need for stitches. Less drastic wounds should be cleansed thoroughly with soap and water, then the edges drawn together with tape; see if the body's healing mechanism can't handle it. If infection should occur, having your doctor culture the wound and treat it with an appropriate antibiotic would be wise. However, infections seldom occur in healthy young women's bodies.

We encourage pregnant women to wear shoes out of doors, as pregnancy increases sensitivity to many things, including bee stings and insect bites.

POSTPARTUM INFECTIONS

Infections of the endometrium, or lining of the uterus, are very rare in natural-childbirth patients. Probably this is related to the fact that no forceps or other instruments are inserted into the uterus, to the decreased need for vaginal exams due to shorter labors, and to the ability of our undrugged experienced mother to tell her attendant when she is going to give birth.

In olden days, this horrible, mother-killing scourge was called "childbed fever." It is characterized by foul-smelling lochia, or vaginal discharge, severe abdominal pain, and fever. There is no effective grandmother treatment, and the physician should be called.

BREAST-FEEDING

A breast infection produces sudden high temperatures, aching, and dizzy feelings, a hot sore spot in the breast; it can be very uncomfortable. The primary cause is exhaustion and inadequate nutrition on the part of the mother along with infrequent nursing. This may cause plugged ducts, which may lead to a breast infection.

The grandmother treatment here consists of nursing often, using the sore breast first. The baby sucks hardest in the first five minutes and this helps to drain the breast. This milk won't hurt the baby at all. Gentle heat, such as is produced by a hot shower, warm bath, or hot-water bottle can be tried for relief. It is also very important for the mother to get lots of rest, plenty of good food, and lots of fluids.

If these simple remedies don't work and the soreness and fever are progressive, antibiotics are indicated, so contact your physician.

FEVER

One of the most effective means the body uses to combat infections, be they viruses or bacteria, is hyperthermia, or fever. The medical myth that drugs should be used immediately, to get fever down as soon as possible, probably interferes with nature's healing process and does more harm than good. Perhaps we should welcome fever as evidence that the body's forces against infection are working.

Excessive fever for long periods of time is a bad sign that the body cannot handle the invaders, and, of course, should be doctor-treated. However, the ordinary initial fever of an infection is normal and should not be countered by chemicals; it is part of the healing process. Fever can be a monitor of the progress of an infection, and its natural disappearance is a good indication that recovery is under way. To suppress it artificially with drugs, like aspirin, fools you into thinking you are getting well when you may not be, and aspirin might be a very harmful drug to babies in the uterus.

HEMORRHOIDS

These tender, often painful bumps in or around the rectal opening are actually varicose veins of the rectum. They sometimes occur in spite of preventive measures (nutrition and Kegels), as sometimes happens in the best of families, as the result of inherited weak veins.

Should simple remedies not work, have your doctor check the problem. He may be able to open a distended vein and let the clot out. Extensive surgery is seldom done in pregnancy, for hemorrhoids usually clear up following birth of the baby.

VARICOSE VEINS OF THE LEGS

If these weak veins break down in spite of preventive measures (see preceding chapter) or if they existed before the pregnancy, then wearing elastic hosiery during pregnancy may be helpful. Consult your doctor about your options.

Should localized sore spots occur, the doctor should check them. Hardly ever are the veins operated on during pregnancy or until childbearing is over, as most will go away afterward.

GENITAL HERPES INFECTION

This has been appropriately called the "leprosy of love" because of its contagious nature and because up to now we have found no cure. Nothing seems to alter its course, so that preventive measures as described in the previous chapter are indicated.

CONSTIPATION

Do not irritate thirty feet of intestine with harsh chemicals to get the last six inches to pass its contents. Make sure there is enough roughage, fruits, and fluids in your diet. Reestablish the gastrocolic reflex by repetition of the above—contact your doctor, if needed.

21

BRADLEY MOMS' PERSPECTIVES AND STORIES

Women have sent us notes, e-mail, and letters telling us how important it was to them to have their husbands present at the birth of their children. Over and over again, women have let us know how vital their husband's role as coach in their births was and how they couldn't have done it without them.

How does a dad make such a difference? How did his role increase the quality of the marriage, closeness of the family, and bonding to the baby? Here are a few notes that moms have shared with us:

We achieved a natural Bradley birth with our third son and it has been the most extraordinary experience of my life. Although my husband was with me for all of our children's births, I did not feel he was as "present" as he was for our Bradley birth. We had a connection that was so powerful that I believe we are still feeling it today, sixteen months later. From our training together to his coaching during the birth, we were an awesome team. The energy from this connection heightened our emotions and positive drive to achieve this beautiful natural start for our baby.

He was my voice and my protector, so all I needed to concentrate on was the birth. He knew exactly what I needed and wanted, and his confident presence gave me added strength through the whole birth. We achieved a short and productive labour with an almost pain-free birth. Although there were other people in the room, they were following *our lead* in contrast to following the way *they* thought the birth should proceed. My husband felt so much more involved in the birth than before and was confident, proud, and happy in his role.

Together we created a life and together we brought him into the world. We've always had the vision and belief system for a natural birth; we just had the wrong tools to achieve it. *Husband-Coached Childbirth,* along with our Bradley natural-childbirth educator, gave us the knowledge, skills, and power to achieve a beautiful natural birth. I have referred many friends and family to this empowering book and I am inspired to one day be a Bradley natural-childbirth educator to help spread the word. I would just like to say one more thing—thank you.—Nikki R.

A husband is so important at the birth and *throughout* the labor. For our second child, my husband came home from work after I had been in labor about three or four hours. Because he hadn't been there, he had a hard time jumping in as coach. He knew how to observe me to see where I was at.

We—he realized that it was time to go . . . Too late and we had the baby at the back door on our way to the car. The coach is another set of eyes and can see and evaluate where Mom is at far better than Mom. So it's good, Very Good to have a husband-coach at the whole labor!—Rachelle M.

Thanks to Bradley, my husband was able to be a part of it all. He went from not wanting to see, to wanting to catch our baby. Even though he didn't get to do that, he still got the joy of doing everything he could to help.—Carrie H.

Having my husband at the birth of our two children was amazing. Just like with anything in our lives, I know that with him, I can do anything. He is a constant source of love and support and I couldn't imagine going through labor without him.

   During my labor, I did not like to be touched or talked to. But I liked having my husband to hold on to (ironically, I could touch him even though I didn't like it the other way around). I held on to him with all that I had, with my entire being. He was my rock. He was my constant. He was my everything in those moments. I can't stress enough how important my husband was. Birth any other way just wouldn't be the same.—Allison K.

Early in our pregnancy, Marcus and I started talking about our expectations for the delivery of our little one. We both expressed interest in natural, unmedicated childbirth. We were shocked to learn in our early pregnancy class, that the epidural rate was higher than 90 percent at the hospital we had chosen to give birth. We knew that if we were serious about giving our baby the best start in life that we would have to look beyond the childbirth classes offered by the hospital.

   I stumbled across The Bradley Method on the Internet and became very curious; I was drawn to the method because of the focus on natural childbirth, the success of the method, but also on the involvement of the husband. Unfortunately, there were no teachers in our area, but I contacted some instructors in our state anyhow. I made a great connection with a Bradley instructor who lived a little over two hours away from our home. Her story with wanting natural childbirth was the same as mine, she provided me with a lot of great information, and invited us to their home and to sit in on a class. After meeting the instructors (a husband and wife team) and sitting through one class, we committed to The Bradley Method.

Labor and childbirth were more physically and emotionally demanding than I could've imagined. Bradley classes never taught us that it would be easy, rather they prepared us for the natural-birth process. My husband was so instrumental in Kalea's birth; from the time we left for the hospital, Marcus never left my side, not even for a moment. I wholeheartedly believe I would not have been able to go through it without his love and support.

Kalea nursed eagerly for at least an hour after she was born and continues in a wonderful nursing relationship with me. She was awake and alert for much of the first twenty-four hours after she was born, and from birth her neck was very strong and she was able to pick up and move her head, unlike the other babies we had seen whose moms chose to have epidurals. We are blessed to have such a happy and healthy little girl, and we believe this was at least in part because she was not under the effects of any medication.

When we look back on Kalea's birth, it is frightening to think of the birth we might have had and the resulting outcomes if we didn't have the information and preparation that the Bradley classes gave us. We are very grateful for our Bradley teachers, the shared experiences of other students, and the members of our birth team who supported our desires for a natural, unmedicated birth. They all had a part in our beautiful Bradley birth, and our beautiful Bradley baby!

Kalea Jean was born at 3:12 a.m., on April 1, in Iowa City, Iowa. She was born a happy healthy baby girl, naturally.—Kara S.

My husband was amazing. I've never needed the kind of mental support that this labor required, yet he was on top of his game the entire time, never emitting an ounce of doubt in our ability to have this baby naturally.

I knew when I was complete and was excited to finally meet the baby we had worked so hard for. About thirty minutes after I had begun pushing, my husband caught our fourth child, a girl, eight pounds, eight ounces, twenty-one inches long.

Our three other children, ages six, four, and two, were there for the birth as well. This was the first birth any of them had seen though we had done lots of prepping with Bradley materials. It was amazing for both us and them! I am a strong advocate now for children at birth and believe it has made our family closer, with deeper intimacy between us all. My two-year-old kept wanting to play with the umbilical cord and called it a "fake worm." The pictures are priceless.—Kathi V.

We did not quite make it to the hospital in time! Instead I gave birth on a blanket on the side of a road! The only people present at the birth were me, Chris, and our daughter. Although we would never choose to have an unattended birth, it was very nice to be left alone to allow nature to take its course. Chris is very proud to have been the one to catch Emily and he is happy that he will be listed on the birth certificate as having delivered her!

For the third time now The Bradley Method has served us well! We felt well prepared for Emily's birth and are very happy with the birth that we could give her.—Susan L.

I was still in some distress. "I'm not in control," I cried. My husband, Chris, ever the sanity check, responded, "No, you're not." I said I thought I needed to be side-lying . . . but I had about one chance to move before everything happened. I knew I needed to, but not how I could manage it. I was stuck. Thankfully, Chris took charge. From his perch behind me, he hooked his arms under mine and just heaved back, pulling me up on top of himself . . . Chris turned, putting me down on my side with him lying on his side behind me, still my strong support. (This must have made poor Chris feel like he was run over by a bus!)

When the baby was born, Chris and I exulted and cried. We'd done it. Our baby, Eleanor Grace (Nora), was here!—Ellen C.

My husband, Jesse, was one of the first fathers allowed to be in the labor and delivery room in Atlanta in 1972. After having two medicated births, in our third pregnancy we sought out a supportive doctor who used *Husband-Coached Childbirth* as his bible for all his dads to read. I was a nervous wreck from problems from the previous drugged deliveries. I had my first natural childbirth the Bradley way with my husband having a more active role in helping me through learning how, by The Bradley Method!

I really clung to my husband, depending on him to see me through all the hard work that was well worth it, and a lot better than the fearful deliveries I had experienced before. We went on to have our fourth . . . Jesse caught our girl himself with the doctor beside him! I depended on Jesse during labor, emotionally and mentally as well as physically, to actively coach me through these births! The hospital staff were supportive, yet I still clung to my experienced husband-coach as if we were the only ones there. Totally lost in his love, his helping me birth our children was more effective than any number of strangers with expertise or drugs that could have been offered.

The love between us as a couple grew with each birth as we worked together to give birth instead of being delivered! I could not have made it without Jesse's helping me! The fears and phobias of birth seemed to disappear as he lovingly gave me undivided attention and love as I gave birth. Thank you, honey!—Bonnie W.

At two-thirty a.m. I woke Steve and told him, "I don't think we'll be going to church today." Steve got up and walked around a little, trying to decide what to do with himself while I stayed in bed on my side. He canned the shower idea and decided to just rub my back instead, which I greatly appreciated.

We continued to time contractions and I decided it would probably be good for me to get up and walk around a little, especially since I didn't feel like lying down anymore. Before I started walking, I figured it would take until midmorning for this baby to come, but once I was up, stuff started to happen!

At three-thirty Steve called Marsena (our midwife)—my contractions were three to four minutes apart and over a minute long. Steve then called my mom and his mom to come over. Contractions got harder very fast and I had a lot of pressure on my bottom.

Steve applied pressure to my back during the contractions. I relaxed through most of my contractions by kneeling in front of the love seat in our bedroom, laying my torso across two pillows on the seat cushions.

I got up and walked between each contraction and returned to the sofa each time one started. Then I had two contractions that were hard—I shook and had tremendous pressure and a desire to push. I was sure I felt the baby actually drop or slip down into the pelvis on the last one.

Mom really helped me through that one by being calm and encouraging me to be calm, too. (It's as though she took a Bradley class—way to go, Mom!)

At this point I was really shaky—my visible sign of transition—even though I was still pretty with it. I don't think I got totally brainless until I was pushing. At any rate, I went over to the bed and Marsena checked me—my only vaginal exam the whole pregnancy—and said I had an anterior lip and a bulging bag of waters. In short, she gave me the okay to push when I felt like it. I lay on my side and Steve encouraged me to take a few more contractions before pushing to really establish readiness (hard to hear from my perspective, but good coaching advice).

I wanted to get into a pushing position and mentioned squatting or something. Marsena suggested all fours, which sounded good to me since I was transitioning into brainlessness. Beth, Marsena, and Steve organized the pads under me while I tried to get onto my hands and knees.

With the next contraction I pushed a little, but not much, while Mom stroked my back and Steve applied pressure (forever applying pressure!) to my back. We worked through two contractions like that and then they set about trying to create a pillow stack for me to rest on during contractions, because I hadn't been off my hands and knees since I got there. What they came up with wasn't all that successful, so I decided to just stick it out where I was.

During the next contraction my water broke, which felt really good—a release of pressure. I joked about ruining my good socks. I sat back on my knees trying to rest. It didn't feel the best, but was my only option. With the next contraction, Molly moved down to crowning and Marsena told me to push gently. I eased up and the pressure and burning were immense. I was shaking badly and Marsena said to only push with the next contraction. We waited and waited and waited for that contraction.

Finally at 5:23 a.m. it came and I pushed Molly out all at one time. I only had a tiny tear, which didn't need repair, and Molly had a knot in her cord, which fascinated Marsena. Molly cried very little and was thickly coated with vernix. She nursed immediately and stayed at the breast for one hour! She was rather unhappy when removed from that position. After the birth of the placenta, Marsena and Beth allowed us to be together with Molly for an hour before doing any checks on her. It was great!

The boys woke up half an hour after Molly was born and came in to see her. Joel was very excited and Asher was upset that it wasn't a boy. They decided to stay up and have breakfast. They actually got to go to church that morning, too.

At the beginning of it all, I never thought Molly would be born so quickly. I was sure labor was going to last a little longer. But all went well and I am tremendously pleased to have been in my house with my family and a few trusted individuals. It was a blessed and Spirit-filled experience for which I will always thank God.—Ginger W.

Todd practically handed out our birth plan to everyone in the maternity ward! It was stated quite clearly that we were not interested in medication of any kind unless certain necessary circumstances deemed so, and only then should they speak to Todd about it first so he could confer with me.

My first "real" contraction was at one a.m. They were about seventeen minutes apart so we were both able to get a semi-decent night of rest. In the morning they started coming about five to seven minutes apart and the nurse really wanted to get things going. She recommended Pitocin quite a few times but we politely declined each time. Finally she referred to our birth plan and asked us to take a walk, take a shower, and do some manual nipple stimulation—all the techniques we had put down that we preferred to do to augment labor. It worked. We took a walk and then I did the stimulation in the shower. The contractions became stronger and closer together almost immediately.

My husband was the best coach I could've hoped for. He attended to my every need and made it possible for me to truly relax my entire body during contractions. Two hours after the OB checked my dilation I felt the uncontrollable need to push. I was at ten centimeters! I pushed for two hours and seventeen minutes and our beautiful baby boy, Rowan, was born.

I couldn't have done it without the incredible support and strength of my husband. He helped me to realize my strength in this natural process. Although there are things I can think of now that I would've done differently and the next time I will probably give birth at home to do away with unnecessary interventions, I am so lucky to have studied The Bradley Method with my husband and that the end result was a healthy mother, baby, and family!—Jodi S.

My contractions began around three-thirty a.m. on the fourth. I had had a few days where I'd have early-morning contractions, but they were sporadic and died out. So I figured I'd keep tabs on these like the others, but I didn't expect anything. Our due date was the fifth, so I knew it could be any day. By four-thirty a.m. John was up and I told him I'd been having contractions. He decided to time them and see if they had any patterns. He had about an hour before he had to leave for work.

By five-thirty a.m. John said we had a pattern and I admitted these contractions were stronger than the ones I had had in earlier days. John had already decided to stay home from work. We decided to call our midwife.

The boys were up and dressed, the cake was made, and the birth tub was full by nine a.m. I read a magazine in between contractions. Our assistant midwife called to check in and say she, too, was on her way. After talking to John a bit, she said the baby sounded like he was OP and I should try a very uncomfortable hands and knees position in fifteen-minute intervals to give him a better chance of turning. I tried it for fifteen minutes, hated it, and decided my body felt better doing my squatting birth dance so I stood up. John agreed I should do what felt best, that I should follow my body's lead.

By nine-thirty a.m., I began to feel pushy at the peak of

contractions. I didn't say anything, but John must have known. He came over to check on me. Conversation was frequently interrupted by contractions. He knows my birth dance well. He looked at the time, close to ten a.m. Where was our midwife? He picked up the phone to call her to see how far away she was and just then she pulled up. I felt better when I saw her car. Now to call Kaye, the lady from church that was coming to help out with the boys. Thankfully, she didn't live far—we couldn't wait any longer. The boys were doing great. They were playing a game on the computer. John was running around trying to keep tabs on me and the boys and still help Paula to get set up.

I went to my room; I knew we were getting close. I went to the bathroom and, boy, did I feel like pushing there! I still didn't say anything—nothing was ready yet. Paula, our midwife, and John were scrambling to set up. When I couldn't resist the push urge with the peaks of the contractions, I told Paula I was feeling pushy.

I was moving faster than she was ready for. Next she checked me, I was at eight centimeters. She checked baby's heartbeat, it sounded good.

I got in the tub. The water felt good. It took the edge off the contractions. John passed the boys off to Kaye and stayed in the room with me. Now I could relax a bit. With everything set up and John staying put, I gave myself permission to let go and push. I had started pushing a bit when I got in the pool. It wasn't until these "pre-pushes" that my mucus plug came out and my water broke.

Once my water broke, I gave about four good pushes and Connor was born, it was 11:14 a.m.—just shy of an eight-hour labor. It was glorious, a little loud, but glorious. No rips, tears, or episiotomies, not even a nuchal cord to contend with. Somewhere in my pushing the boys had entered the room to watch their brother being born. They did a great job and they were very excited to be a part of their brother's birth. I was glad they were there—I was glad John was there.

We had done it. In about a month we had moved to California from Oregon, set up a household, got a midwife, and had a baby. Wow! What a month! Now we could relax a bit and enjoy our new family. It was a great birth day!—Gina B.

It was my second baby and being a Bradley instructor, I was completely prepared . . . I thought. I knew this baby was posterior and had tried everything to get him to turn in the weeks before his birth. When labor began I immediately got in the tub on my hands and knees to try to turn him. Then when labor slowed, my husband and I walked around our neighborhood on and off for a couple of hours. It was getting late in the evening and the contractions were infrequent and not very strong so we both went to bed.

A couple of hours later I knew this was really labor, so I got up and got back in the tub. Matt was by my side and encouraging me to visualize the baby turning. He helped me relax by lighting candles and putting on soothing music. The contractions were not painful, just strong, and I was feeling the pressure in my lower back. When we decided to leave for the hospital, Matt made the transition easy by getting everything ready and being so calm. He was acting like such a pro even though he had only done this once before.

We arrived at the hospital and Matt took care of dealing with the nurses, getting our stuff situated, and getting me ice to suck on, all the while maintaining pressure on my lower back with a rice-filled heating pad. It was the only thing that felt good out of the bath. When I threw up, he got me a pail and cleaned it up, even though he has such a weak stomach that he often throws up while changing a diaper!

We got into the great big hospital tub and he made sure I was comfortable, dimmed the lights, and whispered encouraging words to me for the next few hours. The back labor was intense and I was starting to panic. They had checked me after five hours of hard labor and I was only five centimeters. I was getting overwhelmed and wondering if I could do another five plus hours. He was the ONLY thing that got me through this period of self-doubt. He kept me calm and made me stop clenching my jaw and fists.

Then after an unbelievably hard contraction, I jumped from the tub and my water broke. He was startled and ran like the wind to get the nurse as the baby's head began to crown. After a couple of pushes, the panicked nurse delivered our beautiful baby boy (Aaron Matthew—eight pounds, eight ounces) while my astonished husband shook his head and said he had NO idea I was so close to delivery . . . He said I was too calm and relaxed to be in transition!—Julie O.

My husband was so involved from the beginning. His favorite coaching tool was the emotional signposts. All day I had been leaking amniotic fluid (so I figured). We were visiting his parents when my contractions began. We just visited, watched movies, and I rocked in a chair. I remember really feeling comforted by my dog. He sat on my lap as I rocked and I petted him throughout early labor.

When we decided to go to the hospital, Luke was very careful to check the labor signposts. He made me wait, like a sport coach. In the hospital, he was so supportive; suggesting things like walking, taking a bath, and kept on me to drink water. He was constantly giving me the back rub (and support) I needed. I remember feeling so vulnerable—and here he was, holding my hair back, talking to the nurses for me. He was even using vocalization along with me. He was always right at my side, which is where I needed him most.

When Mia was born, we looked at each other through our tears, with new life, new love, and as a new family.—Anna B.

Taking the Bradley classes really helped improve our marriage and bring us closer to our unborn baby. My husband was wonderful during our birth. I truly feel that I couldn't have done it without him. I was so comfortable with him helping me relax during early labor. During transition he was the person I needed the most. From the Bradley classes he learned to vocalize his feelings toward me and encourage me the entire time. The birth was an amazing experience because my husband was there. I am very thankful that the Bradley classes made the natural birth of my daughter, Madison, an amazing experience for us.—Jodi R.

The thing I appreciated most about having my husband participating in the birth of our daughter was the fact that I knew I could rely on him not to get carried away with his emotions. In everyday life he is very steady and even keeled no matter what, and it is very rare that anything fazes him. So I knew that during labor and delivery his calmness and composure would keep me grounded, just like it always has during every other major event in our lives.—Stephanie N.

BRADLEY DADS' PERSPECTIVES AND STORIES

This book would not be complete without some comments and thoughts from fathers who have coached Bradley births themselves. For further stories check out: www.bradleybirth.com

I have coached my sweetheart through six pregnancies and births. These are the sweetest, most vivid, most unifying, and most defining experiences of our relationship.

We are stronger, more loving, and more committed to each other and to our family because we did this together. There is no experience in this life comparable to witnessing and being part of the birth of one's child.

Helping my wife do it herself, naturally—the way God designed it to happen—has made her dearer to me; and she tells me that I am dearer to her as well. That's something worth having, isn't it?—Steve H.

My wife, Olga, and I have been married since 1974 and that was quite an event in itself, but I digress . . . We are a visually impaired (blind) couple but this has proven to be a minor inconvenience rather than a disability. We've had ten children, most of them were born in Hawaii, some in Alaska, nine out of ten of them were using The Bradley Method and all of them were home births.

The most important things that hit me as a dad (visually impaired) were:

I hear the first cry, boy or girl? (I can usually tell by voice.)
I bond by holding our baby right after birth.
I hear the suckling of the first nursing.
I feel the movements of the baby.
I hear and feel the newborn breaths.
I touch and feel the wet slipperiness of the newborn.
I caress the velvet soft smoothness of the skin after the baby is wiped off.
I smell the fresh scent of a newborn baby.
I can experience and participate during the growth of my family, and be there to support my wife.—Larry K.

HUSBAND-COACHED CHILDBIRTH–WHY?

The concept of the husband as a labor coach or assistant is now widely accepted in society. Many childbirth methods include the father, and hospitals are now much more accommodating to fathers in the delivery room. But, this progress has been a long time in the making; it was 1947 when Dr. Bradley first introduced husbands into the labor process.

Using The Bradley Method, a husband prepares before the labor by studying his wife, practicing with her, talking to her, and learning all he can about labor. When labor begins, the husband must help his wife through the contractions. He helps her to get into a comfortable position, and encourages her to breathe slowly and deeply. He gives her water to drink between contractions, and gives her food if she is hungry. He takes care of any details he needs to, such as taking a bag to the car (if traveling outside the home) and calling the birth attendant. Most importantly, though, he creates the atmosphere of the labor. He talks to his wife. He reassures her that she is doing well, and that she can do it. He minimizes any distractions from people or machines. He puts happy and relaxing images in her mind. He relaxes her with his touch and his voice. He makes sure everything that happens is what is best for his wife and his child.

Why must it be the husband who does this? These duties could be performed by a doctor, midwife, doula, family member, or friend. But the husband is an integral part of the success of The Bradley Method. He is the most important other person to his wife and child. He knows his wife and child (even in the womb) better than anyone else. His wife trusts him more than anyone. And most importantly, he loves his wife and child more than anyone else ever could.

Fathers have a duty and obligation to their families

When a child is preparing to leave the womb, one must consider who might be the most important and qualified people to play a part in this life-altering event. One obvious participant is the mother; the entire process hinges on her involvement. When looking for a partner for her, consider the following questions: Whom did she choose to help create the child? Who else has played the biggest role in the child's life to this point? Who is most likely to be a part of other important moments in the child's life?

A good father will most likely be present for his children's first step, first tooth, first word, first recital or concert, and first sporting event. He will help them eat, sleep, use a toilet, ride a bicycle, read, write, drive, etc. How could he *not* help his child be born? It seems obvious and natural that a father play a role in raising children, so it should be obvious and natural that he has a right and obligation to play an important role in the birth.

Father knows (his wife and child) best

When our child is in the womb, I know when he or she is active, or has the hiccups. I talk to the baby, sing to him/her, and read stories. I know my child's personality from the other side of the womb. When the baby is an extrauterine creature, we know each other already; we are not meeting for the first time.

No one else in the world knows as much as I know about how my wife works. I know when she's happy, sad, worried, angry, tired, uncomfortable, timid, serious, or relaxed. All I need to do is walk into the same room as her, and I can pick up her mood and emotions. Occasionally, she will come to a pause in a sentence, fumbling for a word or name, and I will fill in the blank. She will ask, "How did you know that?" The answer is that I married her, and I know her more intimately than anyone else ever has or will. I know what she likes and dislikes, and how to tell the difference. I know how she feels and thinks.

When my wife is in labor, this is a strong asset. In fact, I can't imagine anyone else trying to get her through it, or myself trying to coach anyone else. It would be like trying to fly the space shuttle; I would press buttons and flip switches in the wrong combinations, and a disaster would ensue. If I had a few days to practice and study, I might be able to avoid a crash. If I had a few months to train, I would probably be able to successfully pilot the craft. Yet there would be an astronaut with years of training, who had flown shuttles before, whose ability would far exceed mine. This is one reason that the husband is the ideal labor coach: no one else has spent the time training that he has. Thus one can deduce that the stronger a marriage or relationship is, the stronger the coach will be.

Trust

I know my wife trusts me implicitly. When she is sick, she wants me to take care of her. When she is not with our children, she wants me to be with them. If we are looking for a new house or car, she wants to make the decision with me. She trusts me, not because I am an expert on any of these subjects, but because I am the most important person in her life. If another person tried to coach her through labor, no matter how skilled he or she was, or how well my wife knew the person, she would never respond as she does to me. She chose to have children with me; that is a sign of a very deep trust. When the stakes are as high as they are in childbirth, when two lives can be changed so drastically, every woman needs to trust in something above all else. Some trust a doctor or midwife, some trust a drug, some trust a friend. My wife trusts me. The stronger the bond of trust between two people, the more effective they can be during labor.

Love

The most important reason for a husband to be a labor coach is the love between him and his wife. Because he loves her and their child more than anyone else does, he has the strongest interest in what is best for them. If a father saw his wife or child in any danger, he would spare no lengths to assure their safety. A father would sacrifice anything for the well-being of his family. Because he loves his wife and child, a Bradley father takes classes with his wife. He reads about labor and birth, and prepares for the event. He makes sure that both mother and baby are well nourished, well rested, and in good shape for labor. The love of her husband is what encourages a mother through labor. He is the most crucial piece to her emotional well-being.

In a loving, trusting marriage, the husband is the best person to coach his wife through labor. The close relationship between husband and wife makes him a good coach, and coaching his wife through labor makes them closer.

Birth is an important event for a family; with the husband as coach, it makes for a strong, caring, loving, and healthy family.—Christopher L.

OUR BIRTHING EXPERIENCE

Our birthing plan was complete. It was filled with our wishes and intentions. We tried to both clearly communicate our wants and do so in a respectful way. We did not want our medical team to feel disrespected, defensive, or unimportant.

Several copies were made to pass out to all medical personnel. When we arrived at the hospital it was important for us to distribute it to a couple of nurses right away because my wife's water had broken before we had arrived and they were quick to discuss inducing labor.

After we had our initial testing and so forth, we were moved to the labor and delivery room. Once we arrived there and my wife was settled, I asked the nurse how she would like me to get a birthing plan to each participating medical-team member. It was her idea to set some copies at the nurses' station.

Our birthing process, from the beginning through second stage, was just about ideal. Our personal experience was seamless and we felt comfortable and confident in our natural approach using The Bradley Method. However, our medical staff was neither comfortable nor confident.

When my wife had dilated to about three or four centimeters, she began to focus. This stage of labor my wife was going through was perceived as painful to the medical staff, perhaps because it usually is in their unnatural circumstances.

As a result of perceived pain, a nurse walked through the door into our room and subtly mentioned that she had some Pitocin just in case we thought we wanted to speed up labor. I was surprised about this because our birth plan clearly mentioned we were open to medication only in critical circumstances and all discussion regarding medication should go through me first and in private, away from my wife who was busy concentrating and had no room for erroneous distractions. I figured this particular nurse just hadn't seen the plan. No big deal, I figured, she'll catch on.

A second nurse entered the room an hour or so later mentioning she was bringing in some painkillers, located conveniently next to my wife's head, just in case the pain got too bad.

After five or so of these experiences, I had to intervene. It was my time as the coach to maintain the proper environment for my wife. I asked the nurse to speak with me outside the room. I asked her if she would gather up another nurse or two, anyone who may be in our room at any time, because I had a very important message for them. At this point, I respectfully yet firmly explained our plan as it related to medication. It was important for me to not beat around the bush as I knew my wife was in a vulnerable position. I emphasized we were not opposed to medication with the exception of normal circumstances. I reassured them I was thankful and recognized their concern.

From this point forward the medical team did a great job of respecting our wishes. My wife and I had a successful birthing experience and we feel truly blessed with the process, the outcome, and our wonderful baby.—Todd S.

When we first took Bradley Method classes, we knew that both of us wanted to be involved in the birth of our baby . . . but we had no idea how important that would be! The labor with our son, Kyle, ended up lasting fifty-one hours. During that time, as my wife's labor coach, I found myself working to keep in tune to her needs and taking care of everything before she asked. The things we learned in class and practiced were very useful. I rubbed her back when it was sore; made sure she had sips of juice and snacks, and according to her, was the "rock" that she needed to get her through the most challenging, but rewarding, experience of our lives. I lost count of how many times I praised her, walked beside her up and down the hall, and labored with her in the birth tub! I was very tired at the end, but when she kissed me and said thank you, and told me she could never have done it without me, it was all worth it.:)—Michael U.

When my wife and I found out we would be having a baby, it took little time to discover we both wanted to have a natural childbirth. To us, it didn't make any sense to take any unnecessary risks during labor and delivery, and we wanted our baby to have the best start in life possible. For me personally, maybe a little selfishly, I wanted the birth of my first baby to be an experience, not just an event.

Although we knew what we wanted, my wife wasn't sure if we would be able to accomplish our goals without training. Being a man and in the medical field, my first thought, of course, was that we'd "figure it out." After talking about it and researching the possibilities, we decided that we would try The Bradley Method.

Unable to find a Bradley instructor in our area, we decided we would go to one session with an instructor about two and a half hours away and see what it was like. Sitting through one class, we knew we had found what we were looking for.

Now that the joyous event has come and gone, my wife and I are so glad we completed the Bradley training. They say that knowledge is power, and we believe that the training gave us the power to make our birth experience successful and unique to us. I would not have been nearly prepared to deal with the stress, anticipation, and anxiety of labor, nor been able to assist my wife effectively without the training from Bradley classes.

The knowledge of the birthing process including staging and normal processes was invaluable. The guided-relaxation practice was also helpful. Most importantly,

seeing and speaking with couples that have actually completed training and had successful births was inspiring and
reassured us that we were capable, prepared, and that we
were making the right decision.

My wife had been having Braxton-Hicks contractions
during the final months of pregnancy, but on Thursday,
something was different. By morning, the contractions
were getting more intense, but were not consistent, so we
thought it could be hours or even days until the "real
thing." At about ten a.m., I got a call at work. "Are you
planning on coming home soon?"

When I got home, I saw that my wife had cleaned our
house, done laundry, and been working on some things for
her office, but was still having contractions.

At nine-thirty p.m. I called the hospital and told them
that my wife's contractions were down to three to five minutes apart, and they told us to come in.

We arrived in the labor and delivery department a little
after ten p.m. I remember a strange feeling as we walked to
the desk past a room where a woman was giving birth to
twins. I glanced toward the room and could see the tubes
and pump from the mother's epidural. It reinforced what I
wanted. I wanted this birth to be what it should be, a life-
changing experience between a wife and husband.

The doctor on call was less than receptive to our birth
plan. I knew my wife was disappointed. I knew that this
was the reason we took The Bradley Method training. No
matter what was happening around us, we knew what we
did and did not want. The Bradley Method training helped
us stay focused on that and confident.

After hours of labor and some concern about the baby's
heart rate, my wife entered into what I would call a trance-
like state. I guess you could call it transition. I remember
the most extraordinary love-reaffirming, heart-to-heart
connection as I was able to have her refocus her thoughts,
calm down, and not fight the pain.

I think because the phrase "urge to push" was used so

much by everyone explaining how contractions felt to signal delivery, we didn't realize what was happening at first. Even though the doctor had just checked my wife moments before, the nurse checked my wife again and announced that she was fully dilated and ready to deliver. My wife looked at me and asked if she was supposed to push or not. I asked her if she felt the "urge" to push. She said no, but discovered that when she did push, there was much less pain.

One more little push, and as quick as the delivery started, it was over. Kalea was placed on my wife's belly as we had wanted and wiped down. In all the excitement, I nearly forgot to take pictures.

There I was with my wife and brand-new baby girl. I couldn't believe what had just happened. It was the most rewarding and fulfilling moment I have ever felt.

It was like a rite of passage, a life-changing, bonding event in the life of a man and a woman. In my heart I don't think it would have been nearly as meaningful if drugs were used. I am so thankful for The Bradley Method. It gave me the confidence and determination to coach my wife through the most amazing process of life.—Marcus S.

I have always been awed by the human body and the beauty of its creation. This is probably what led me into the field of health care. But it wasn't until the birth of our first child that it all became very real to me. While that experience was great, somewhere inside we felt like it could have been better. After our second child was born, with the "help" of a very old-fashioned doctor, we knew that it definitely could be better.

At the time I was in chiropractic college, taking advanced obstetrics and gynecology and working on a research paper. (My instructor was a medical doctor and needless to say we had a very different view on how childbirth should be.) We continued searching for better alternatives for our own births. It wasn't until after our third (birth center) and fourth (home) births that we found The Bradley Method. Even though we had had great experiences with both of these births and weren't even expecting at the time, we decided to sign up for a series of classes. This was what we had been looking for.

With our next two pregnancies (three births—the last were twins) we again took Bradley classes. Some might wonder why, with all the education and experience, we would continue taking classes. I feel that you cannot be over prepared and new information is available from time to time, it made sense. Plus we enjoyed the time together to talk, practice, and prepare for the birth of each child.

What I like about The Bradley Method of husband-coached childbirth is the vast amount of information as well as the consistent reminders to eat right, exercise, and do relaxation. At first I didn't know if I agreed with eating all that protein, but after the birth of our six- and seven-pound twin boys, I knew that was the reason we were able to have a healthy, natural, full-term birth. Also the fact that most of the instructors have experienced firsthand natural childbirth and given the long proven track record, I haven't found a better way to prepare for childbirth.

I would highly recommend The Bradley Method to anyone committed to having a natural birth or at least open to exploring the possibility. Thanks for letting me share.—Todd W.

My being active in our childbirth is the highest form of lovemaking that I have ever experienced or will ever experience.—Roger C.

Both our daughter, Justine Hannah, and our son, Cory David, were born after my wife and I took Bradley classes. We strongly believe that birth is a normal physiological event in the life of a woman. We had read widely, interacted with many health professionals, and taken tours of hospital facilities. This gave us valuable perspectives on the available options, and reinforced our belief in a natural-birth process without unnecessary drugs or other interventions. Bradley classes provided an enormous amount of useful and well-organized sources of information, with effective techniques for natural childbirth. The coach was correctly portrayed as a critically important part of the birth process.

As a trained coach, I felt indescribable joy at the natural childbirth of our daughter and son without the use of any significant medical interventions. My wife, Eva, came through with "flying colors" before, during, and after both births. The emotions that came across at those moments are difficult to accurately recount, but involved an experience of the generational chain.

Directly participating and coaching my wife during the births were the most moving experiences of my life. It helped to form an unbreakable bond with my children that previous generations of fathers rarely had the opportunity to feel. I am truly grateful for being able to have really "been there" in a helpful and fully participatory way. Every minute of study and practice helped to prepare for those moments.

Please continue the great work, and encourage mothers and fathers to be full partners in the birth experience. There is nothing like it in the world!—Jerry F.

It was important to be able to share in the emotional joy, not only in the moment of birth, but throughout the whole labor. It was also important to me to be my wife's active supporter and partner.

The neatest part also was just being able to see the miracle of birth. I see birth now, as God's gift to us, God slowly opening His hands as if to say, "Here is the baby you've waited so patiently for, to take care of and raise." —Michael C.

It was important to have a healthy birth for my baby and my wife. Sharing in the bonding experience, both physically and psychologically with Linda, throughout labor and birth. Being that connected allowed me to react accordingly.

Being the first person to touch our baby was such an emotional buildup. That went beyond physically being there. It was total emotion.—Eric P.

Being with my wife was very important to me, coming from a culture where the man doesn't do that. It was very important being with my wife during the whole labor from start to end. Being there to support her, she'll know you're there, and with the educational awareness I learned from class, witnessing the whole thing was the greatest experience. We recommend Bradley to most of the pregnant couples we meet. It was a super way to do it.—Christopher S.

It was very important to me. It meant being part of the whole thing. If not I would have felt unfulfilled. The thought of her in another room going through that would have made me crazy. It makes my love for Laura close. Of course, seeing my baby come out made it very neat, it made Steven real instead of just popping into my life.—Erick W.

It was extremely important. I felt I didn't have an option whether to do it or not, it was my responsibility, we both made the baby. It was a big support for Tina. It was a lot more exciting than I thought it would be. It exceeded my expectations. I think fathers should be required to take part in the birth.—Chuck G.

First and foremost, I was at the birth to give support to my wife. I knew she needed me, and I wasn't about to let down the most important person in my life.

The actual moment of birth was the bonus. However, had it not been for the preparation I received from our Bradley instructor, I would have merely been an observer, rather than a major contributor.

Looking back, I see now that being a trained coach at my daughter's birth was the highest expression of love I could have given her and my wife. I am forever grateful for the precious gift that God gave us.—David P.

Husband-coached childbirth was important to me because that's the total picture for our family unit. Everyone should be there! I wouldn't have missed it for the world. —Sunny G.

We don't have a lot of medical technology here (Alaska) so we need to try to prevent things from happening. If someone gets into The Bradley Method early enough, then they can remain independent and not worry about having to be flown out [to Seattle or Anchorage]. The Bradley Method is compatible with the rugged individualism that is the Alaskan image. One doesn't need lots of technology to have a baby.—Dave S.

I was very involved throughout my wife's pregnancy and was at the births of both my daughters. Being at the births allowed me to bond right away with my daughters and to create an attachment that I see now has helped our relationship as a family. Being at their births wasn't even a question; as their father, where else would I have been? —Paul W.

It prepared me emotionally for the most important event in my life, the birth of my daughter. Thanks to The Bradley

Method, we learned how important it was to be educated on nutrition, exercise, pain-relief therapy, etc., from the very start. I mean months and months ahead of time. It also gave me some valuable insight about being polite but assertive with medical professionals. And because it emphasizes the importance of the husband, it made me feel like I was as important as the doctor and nurses in helping my wife bring a beautiful, healthy baby in the world. She certainly appreciated my competent and confident support.

Our daughter scored a 10 on the Apgar scale—and she's been healthy ever since. Although my wife experienced some pain during labor, she refused painkilling medication because we wanted our daughter to come into the world alert and energetic. This program motivated us to go "natural" and, as a result, my daughter will benefit for the rest of her life.—Mike S.

Prior to the birth of our first child three years previously, my wife and I worked toward the goal of having a natural childbirth. Unfortunately, despite our Lamaze classes and practice, we ended up with an epidural and finally C-section.

In looking for help with our second child we were introduced to The Bradley Method. In learning The Bradley Method all the obstacles we had encountered in our first birth were addressed and answered. We found out the problems we had were normal and could probably be overcome with some basic natural techniques.

On the birth of our second child, the same problems did, in fact, arise again, but were easily overcome, and we had a wonderful and I daresay relatively easy birth. As an interesting and important point here, after the second hour of pushing the doctor was literally tapping his foot waiting on our approval for a C-section. . . . I kid you not.

The experience was without a doubt one of the most fulfilling in my lifetime! It also points out that while modern medicine is wonderful and in childbirth certainly necessary in certain extreme instances, The Bradley Method proves beyond any doubt that nothing delivers babies more efficiently, safely, or enjoyably than Mother Nature. (I would be honored if all or part of this experience could be used in any way to further the awareness of The Bradley Method.)—Brian D.

When my wife, Elaina, and I found out we were expecting our second child, we immediately began discussing our desires for the birth experience. After the birth of our first child, Greg, we had some regrets about things that happened, and we wanted to avoid those things with this delivery. Our first step was to enroll in Bradley classes. The second step was to choose a doctor and hospital carefully. We wanted to have a say in what happened through the pregnancy and at the birth, something we didn't have with Greg.

Even though we wanted better this time, seeing my first son born was a great experience and he is a wonderful child, but the doctor acted like he was in charge and he put pressure on us to follow standard procedures.

In January, we had our second son, William, and the experience was so much better the second time. As a result of our diligent preparation, we had an experience that forever brought our family even closer together. We even had Greg, who was two at the time, present at the birth and he has been so close to his baby brother from the first day. William seemed to bond immediately with each family member in the delivery room, and we have all been close to him from the first day. It was an experience I wouldn't have missed for anything and I strongly recommend that fathers take an active role in the births of their children. It can be a joyous occasion that will pay big dividends for the whole family.—Brian M.

Rosie's birth was the most beautiful experience I've ever been involved in.—John Y.

In the era of the Men's Movement I can think of no better way to begin a close bonding relationship with one's child than to share the experience of childbirth through husband-coached childbirth.—Doug M.

It is hard to relate my emotional reactions to such an event, but being in that quiet room with the dim dawning light and just the three of us being involved was what can certainly be called the miracle of birth. It was a highly climactic experience. As we drove home that same afternoon with our brand-new daughter, we felt we had shared the ultimate intimacy. That's the feeling I would urge every loving, expecting couple to strive for.—Keith D.

I was by my wife Laurie's side during every moment that our first two children were being delivered by cesarean section. Those experiences, I now realize, were more Laurie's than ours. Of course, in certain obvious ways all pregnancies and births are a unique blessing to women that men will never truly understand, but that is not what I intend to express.

I remember being in the operating room with my little mask, a loose-fitting bonnet, a gown, and paper slippers on and how it gave me the feeling of being privileged, as if I was being treated by the doctors and nurses with special consideration somehow as I watched them take our children by knife from the precious intrauterine intimacy of their mother's body. Looking back now I realize just how much those events were sweeping us along in their own way.

Being the second of nine children had afforded me some insight into pregnancy and childbirth. I witnessed my mother and learned from her while she was pregnant with my younger brothers and sisters. I already understood pregnancy and childbirth was not simply a waiting period for the father and I was determined not to offer only an occasional pat or rub on Laurie's growing abdomen with adoring eyes as the extent of my involvement. I have to admit, though, that I didn't realize what the full weight of my involvement was meant to be during those months of Laurie's first two pregnancies.

Although Laurie and I had sought information to be prepared for our first two children within the whole realm of pregnancy and childbirth, so we thought, I believe we were partakers of a common pool of available information that kept us at a lesser degree of effectiveness to call the shots ourselves than we could have been. We came to learn later that we had overlooked studying key elements of pregnancy and childbirth that The Bradley Method classes exposed us to. There were several concerns to examine beyond the biological factors alone.

Exposure to The Bradley Method had the sobering effect of snapping fingers before entranced parents. Our eyes were opened to realize more fully how much influence we had in determining how our upcoming birth experience would unfold and how often couples have been swept along as we had been by the direction of the medical community, impersonal typewritten advice from faceless authors, special-interest-group propaganda or fate.

As our Bradley Method instructor related more and more pregnancy and childbirth truths to us, my experiences as a father-of-three-to-be changed dramatically. I began to feel the weight of worry over unanswered questions and the feeling of ineptness lift from my shoulders and I knew that I would not have to wait for the crown of my fatherly pride and joy to be placed on my head at the moment my child was born. I could feel it above my brow during our first classes.

I was a father to my third child before I really was a father. I was quickened and qualified by participating in The Bradley Method classes to fulfill all the functions of a husband-coach. A richly rewarding position in more ways than I can adequately express.

When our daughter, Moriah, was born by vaginal birth after two cesarean sections, I had been caring for her long before she felt my touch. And I did so in front of the hospital staff and not peering around them.

I believe we are to strive earnestly to become the best stewards we can be, and best Mommy and Daddy, too, of the most important little creations our Maker has placed in our charge—our children. Though my Christian faith is bedrock, the familiar serenity prayer includes a request for wisdom and the ability to exercise it. I'm very thankful that The Bradley Method exists and is available to dispense some of the wisdom we all need to manage pregnancy and childbirth.—Miguel G.

I was really glad to be a part of my daughter's birth on March 20. My wife really wanted to do a water birth but she was too relaxed, so we moved to a stool birth, which was how my daughter was born. I liked all the different options and it made me feel like I was part of the birth, not just pacing in the waiting room handing out cigars. My wife did a great job and I was very proud of her and how well she handled it.—Joshua H.

The most important reason for the father to be at his child's birth is to be at his child's birth. The father is a great comfort to the mom with whom he is intimate. He also works as a buffer for the mother, controlling lights, music, nurses, questions, and anything else from the outside that can intrude on the serenity you are trying to create.

Our second birth was at home. The peaceful environment was easier to establish. I was free to just observe more. But because of the lack of attendants, I was free to whisper to my wife (I did that during labor). I carried the baby from room to room. Most of all, do not miss this once-in-a-lifetime experience for each baby.—Micha M.

WHY IS IT IMPORTANT TO GET BRADLEY'S HUSBAND-COACHED CHILDBIRTH TRAINING?

As a husband and soon-to-be father, The Bradley Method training is incredibly important. In our culture most men never get any training in childbirth and/or parenting. Many girls practice parenting skills throughout childhood, but boys often don't get the opportunity to practice caring for others as children, and often enter marriage and then have to rapidly learn those missing skills.

GI Joe and Power Rangers don't train you to be a kind, loving, and informed husband and/or parent. We understand the birds and the bees and biology of sex, but our educational system has neglected the fact that husbands/lovers need to know exactly what to expect during childbirth in real and concrete terms, and how to best support, coach, and care for their partners during the pregnancy and delivery.

It is impossible to make intelligent, informed decisions as a couple if both of you don't know the different things that can happen during the pregnancy and birth, and the benefits and consequences of each of your possible choices. The training you will receive on husband-coached childbirth through The Bradley Method classes will prepare you for your new role as a better, more supportive, more knowledgeable, more skilled partner for your wife, and prepare you to take on your new role as father.

Caring for your wife through childbirth will strengthen your bond to her, and her bond to you. It will help both of you be ready to care for your new baby. In our world today, there are very few occasions that a husband can be the "knight in shining armor" for his wife. Taking good care of your wife through her pregnancy and birth lets you perform in that role.

This year our fifth baby was born, and she is beautiful and perfect. We have taken childbirth classes with each of the five pregnancies. Each of the births of our children has been different, and we have learned more about pregnancy and birth with each child. Don't skip taking childbirth classes just because you and your wife have had a baby before. The next delivery may be completely different with different problems and solutions.

Couples need to take the classes again to be reminded of the "right things" to do during this pregnancy, and to prepare for each special and unique delivery and baby. So many things are going on in your life during the pregnancy that it is easy to forget to do the simple and easy things that you both should be doing to get ready for the birth. Taking the classes keeps you on task, working on good nutrition, exercise, stretching, all while learning the information necessary to prepare for the birth.

The childbirth classes we took for our first three children were not The Bradley Method. We found that the instruction in The Bradley Method gave us the additional information and training that we wanted. Most of the other childbirth classes we have taken only lasted four to six weeks.

The Bradley Method's twelve-week curriculum gives the additional time needed to go into much more depth on relaxation techniques to help deal with and avoid excess pain during the birth. We learned about nutrition to keep both the mother and baby healthy, exercises and stretching that will help the mother during the delivery and afterward for her recovery, learned about the pros and cons of the various procedures and medications that may be offered during the pregnancy and delivery, and much more.

While attending The Bradley Method classes and thinking about how the other births went, we discovered the reasons for some of the problems we had had during the other deliveries. My wife had terrible leg cramps during labor. In the Bradley training we learned that the "breathing" that we had learned in our earlier classes had her hyperventilating . . . muscle cramps are a consequence.

After putting the information together, it all made sense. With the Bradley births my wife didn't have the problem of the painful cramps.

There is an old quote that states, "Knowledge is power." Entering into parenthood, dealing with pregnancy and childbirth, you need all the power you can get. We train for marathons, we train for sports, we train for our careers. It is now time to train for our vocations as husbands, lovers, and fathers. The knowledge and skills you will learn in your Bradley Method childbirth classes will help you get started training on being a better husband and father with the power that comes with knowledge.—David W.

23

PHOTOGRAPHING A BIRTH

My parents flew to Denver, Colorado, so I could be born naturally with my father present at my birth. I'm James Hathaway and I have the distinct privilege of being the birth that started the Bradley educational program. I have been at countless births and my photographs have appeared in international magazines, books, newspapers, etc. I have made lots of videos and am an award-winning photographer.

THE PSYCHOLOGY OF CHILDBIRTH PHOTOGRAPHY

Personally, I have been going to births my entire life, starting at just months old. Births are a beautiful, magical experience that everyone has been part of. Whether you realize it or not, we were all born, and someone was there. It is important for humans and animals to see and experience birthing. We learn from watching, and grow from the experiences that we all have. My father is a photographer, so as soon as I could hold a camera I started taking pictures of everything, including the births my mother took me to.

It was easy to realize that a birth is a once-in-a-lifetime event that can never be captured again. This mom may have another baby and have another birth, but it will never be the same as the one you are currently photographing.

THE CAMERA

First consider what kind of camera you feel comfortable with. You may have a camera you love and know how to use. If this is the time to buy a new camera, you might want to consider one with the latest features, but weigh the advantages versus the cost. Inexpensive cameras may not take a picture as quickly or may not have a flash and cannot be used in a variety of situations. I have used cameras ranging from cheap to professional and, to tell the truth, sometimes the pocket cameras are much easier and simpler to have with you and can take incredible pictures.

Cameras come in a variety of sizes, from ones that fit in your pocket to ones that seem to have so many accessories they overshadow the camera itself. Some can be so heavy they need a tripod. The popular small cameras have a lot of features that make them very practical. Memory (cards or sticks) have for the most part replaced film and have tremendous capacity, giving you the ability to store hundreds of shots on each device.

Some cameras have steady shot, which compensates for movement, yours or whatever you are standing on while taking the shot. Some have night vision (infrared), which could be used in a darkened room. Some can shoot rapid shots (one after another), which helps to capture a burst, two or three or more pictures at a time. Some cameras can go underwater, which could be useful if you were attending a water birth or unfortunately standing too near when the bag of waters breaks. Remember that it could be used later when on a trip to the ocean or during inclement weather.

CAMERA SENSITIVITY (ASA OR ISO SETTING)

Some cameras have the ability to shoot with less light, but this increases the overall grain or pixelization of the image (decreasing clarity). For instance, if you take a picture you might notice that it looks great on the screen of the camera but, when blown up (increasing the size of the image) it will become pixelated, or very grainy. Sometimes this is considered artsy and has a certain flair about it. You will need to balance this idea and decide which is most important to you.

If you were taking a portrait you would want to have the highest resolution to have the greatest detail. On the other hand, if you were taking a picture of a sign that you just need to read you could forgo some quality for a smaller picture.

Every camera is different. Do you need a flash or does it come with the camera? What kind of lighting will be in the birthing room? Find somewhere you can take pictures with that kind of lighting now, so you can see what happens. Spend a little time and think about what you want to capture, but also be flexible enough to capture those unexpected shots.

ANGLES

If you shoot from the side instead of head-on you can achieve more discreet images. A leg can be a great prop in helping screen private parts, changing to the true focus on the baby.

Also it is important to try shots from high or low, left or right, and so on. Changing your position or that of the camera can dramatically alter the composition of the shot and can possibly give you that outstanding shot you've always wanted.

LENSES

Cameras either come with a fixed (attached) or interchangeable type lens. For birthing situations having a wide angle lens is extremely beneficial due to the small spaces and closeness that cannot be compensated for by backing up farther into the corner of a room. Learn the wideness of your lens by taking pictures and see just how much image can be obtained with its current lens. If you have a camera with a changeable lens, you may want to invest in getting a wide angle lens, or adaptor.

LIGHTING

Keep in mind your lighting choices. Natural, incandescent, flood, spot, or a variety of other choices. Cameras today can usually be used without having to add lighting.

Available lighting is the simplest. Adding lights or changing the lighting conditions can easily enhance your images. The easiest and less invasive option is to turn on an extra light or use bounced lighting.

BOUNCED LIGHTING

Bounced lighting is taking a strong light source and pointing it up into the corner of a room and using the ceiling to change that light source into a giant diffused lighting system. The advantage of diffused lighting is to help soften and limit the amount of shadows. Picture a white or light-colored cloudy day. . . . This is nature's natural way of giving us diffused lighting. On a sunny day you get harsh shadows. On a cloudy day, everything will have a softer shadow effect or no shadowing at all.

Think about the birthing environment. During labor there may need to be reduced or no lighting, making it difficult or nearly impossible to get a good picture. Realize that flash photography can be distracting and cause a laboring woman extra stress. Be careful and take into consideration the necessity for a noninvasive birthing environment.

On the flip side . . . During the pushing stage lights are usually turned up and the addition of flash photography is hardly noticed. Newborns have been living in a reduced light environment so be cautious and give them a break between taking flash pictures. Some flashes can be angled up so the light can bounce off a surface instead of flashing directly into eyes.

Be creative, have fun, and don't let this unique opportunity pass you by. Every birth is unique and a wonderful opportunity to capture a once-in-a-lifetime situation.

MOVIES

Capture a kind of time record of the birth. Get shots that help tell the story. Think about what you, and others, would want to see. Sometimes you might have to plan ahead and sometimes set the stage. It's great to use natural settings, but you can also clean up (not capture in your angle something that detracts from the subjects) by shooting in another direction to enhance what you are able to record.

BLEND IN

If you are the one shooting this birth, remember a photographer should not get in the way of the birthing process! When I go to a birth it is discussed with the couple that at any time they are uncomfortable or just don't want photos taken at that time . . . Then by all means, I step out and do everything possible to stay out of the way. Let the laboring woman have whatever she needs to feel comfortable and in control of the birthing environment. You could be called back in at any moment.

I am honored and find seeing a birth to be a very rewarding experience. Talking ahead of time about the shots the couple desires helps to give me ideas and a kind of map of what and what not to do. Sometimes I'm asked not to take any picture until pushing has begun. Other times candid photos are desired. It really depends on what is going on with this birth. Try and find out if people are camera shy or big hams. Some people love to have their picture taken while others cringe at the notion.

COMFORT LEVELS

I find that it can be difficult to get certain shots. It can be hard to, in essence, direct the subject matter and can be inappropriate. Asking for a smile or look in this direction can be difficult at times. So you need to be aware of posed shots versus just getting those natural gems that come your way. Asking for simple changes do influence and truly can make the shot. Example: asking people to get closer to the baby for a picture. Look at what others have done in magazines or books or family albums. These are great resources and help to get those creative juices flowing.

EQUIPMENT

The most important things to remember in taking pictures are the film or media card (memory), camera, and charged batteries. Nothing can be worse than forgetting any of the above and just not having any options. Having more than one of everything is always a good idea.

How about extra memory? Have you thought about the software you need on your computer to download these pictures, edit them, put them into albums, and send e-mail copies to friends and relatives shortly after birth? A cherished memory could be that mobile-phone picture you send to the grandparents seconds after the birth.

PRACTICE

Next . . . start taking pictures. Lots of pictures! Remember that it is easier to delete some pictures rather than roll back time. Whether it's your baby or someone else's baby, every picture you take is time sensitive and the photo opportunity will not be exactly the same ever again. Become comfortable and aware of the settings and functions of all your equipment. Don't wait until the birth-day to take your new camera out of the box; become familiar with how to use it well in advance. Take lots and lots of pictures in a variety of conditions so you will be prepared to take pictures like it was second nature to you.

PLAN

What kind of pictures do you want to have, and to what extent should people go to achieve them? Do you mind flash photography or strong lighting? If your wife is pregnant, then these are pictures you will show your baby, toddler, child, teenager about how excited you were being pregnant and expecting this new baby. These pictures prove your love and how much you are willing to do to make sure this baby has the best possible start in life.

If you are extremely modest, realize that with photo software and cropping an image, you might wind up with an edited picture that may be your favorite and most cherished image.

PRE-LABOR PHOTO OPPORTUNITIES OR SHOT LIST

Bradley childbirth classes
Preparing for the birth
Shopping
Pictures of the mom and dad during pregnancy
Tummy photos
Profile shots
Maternal images
Expressions with views of the belly
Other family members before the arrival
Walking and exercising
Eating and drinking
Making room in your home for the new baby
Talking
Pictures of where you live
Where the baby will be born
Clothes for the new baby
Mom and Dad holding hands
Add your own favorite shots

WHO'S YOUR PHOTOGRAPHER?

Who is going to take pictures during labor and birth? Dad can take some pictures but his primary role is that of a father who coaches his wife in labor. This means he may be busy rubbing her back, holding her up, or just talking her through a contraction. Dr. Bradley said: "A husband should be man enough to finish what he starts!" It is not only important for the father to be present and the primary coach, but being at a birth can be beneficial for other family and friends as well. The chance to observe a birth is the chance to watch a miracle—the miracle of life.

You might want to ask a family member or friend to take pictures for you. It needs to be someone whom the mom feels comfortable with and is willing to be there at all hours and leave especially during transition if the mom wants.

LABOR/BIRTH PHOTO SHOT LIST

Pictures of the couple early in labor
Tummy photos
Profile shots
Walking in labor
Family waiting for the birth
Labor contractions
Leaning into the coach
Talking
Relaxing
Facial expressions
Hands
Coaching
All attendees working
Pushing
Discreet images
Non-discreet images, which can always be deleted or
    cropped (discuss ahead of time what you are most com-
    fortable with)
Baby emerging

Baby out and being positioned on Mom
Mom and baby (first time)
Mom, baby, and Dad (first time)
Family (first time)
Nursing
Hands of baby with Mom, Dad, siblings, etc.
Baby looking around
Hands and feet
Placenta
Cutting cord
Weighing
Length
Exam
Mom drinking orange juice
Walking (first time for Mom)
Dad and baby
Others and baby
If beanies (caps) or booties or blankets used, ask if they can
   be removed for better pictures
If home, hanging out at home
If hospital or birth center, getting into car, leaving
Arriving home
Meeting family and friends
Babies grow quickly . . . picture at one hour, day, week,
   month, year
Special events
And, of course, once a year on their birthdays

BONDING

Bonding is crucial for setting the stage of a lifelong bond and commitment to the newborn and family. By partaking and participating, a bond is formed that is stronger and more sustainable than one where you are introduced to this new family member through a pane of glass. Photos are a beautiful way to take an event and instantly freeze it in time. A lot of women will forget many details during the birthing process. Photos and videos can be truly cherished recorded memories and a way to strengthen the family bond. It is a real honor to be present and photograph the event.

Think Pulitzer, Oscar, Emmy!!! And just have fun!

24

DAD'S COACHING TIPS

The role of the coach is a very important one. It is a great responsibility that results in great rewards. The support and interest in pregnancy, birth, and life are things a mother needs and appreciates. This book, along with Bradley classes, will help prepare the coach so he can execute this responsibility with confidence and knowledge. The keys to good coaching in pregnancy and birthing are: support, relaxation, nutrition, exercise, and knowledge.

SUPPORT

Being there 24/7 makes a huge difference. Let her know that this is a team effort. This is the new generation conceived between the two of you. It is your lineage from generations before you. It may be one of the most remembered and enjoyed events in your life. Get ready!

RELAXATION

She needs to know that when she is tense or stressed out, you are there to help her. Remember that relaxation is the key to labor. It is a skill. When relaxation is practiced on a daily basis for at least twelve weeks it can become a powerful pain-management tool in labor and life.

NUTRITION

What could be more important than nutrition for the growth and development of your baby and its mother getting ready for birth? Make it your responsibility to see to it that this mother not only has the food she needs, but your enthusiastic support.

EXERCISE

Training, in an athletic way, can make a big difference when it comes down to the stamina to labor and give birth. Birthing is like running a marathon or climbing a mountain. Help her and join her in the pregnancy exercises and stamina exercises she enjoys and needs.

KNOWLEDGE

This is where classes come in. Taking Bradley twelve-week classes helps to prepare you for this amazing event. We cover the entire birth process, and there should be no surprises even if something unique arises and you need to be flexible. Learn from class, books, and other dads, so you know the course.

WHAT OTHER PEOPLE MAY SAY

The stories of childbirth pain, suffering, and fear go on and on. Very few people have seen a trained couple give birth naturally—

and experience the joy, excitement, and pride in accomplishing what they started out to do.

Most women do not know how to give birth, and men do not know how to help them. The same goes for labor. Women have no idea how to deal with or handle contractions—and they fear the pain they have heard about. Unfortunately bad stories are repeated seven to one over good stories, and perhaps more than that in reference to childbirth.

The truth about birthing is that every single person on the face of this earth has an amazing family history of generation after generation of successful, drug-free birthing, or you would not be here. Your mother may have taken drugs when you were born, she might even have been a cesarean and your grandmother may have taken drugs when your mother was born. But the chances are your great-grandmother gave birth naturally, and *her* mother gave birth naturally, and on and on. Each generation passed down the knowledge of how to birth until the 1900s when birth was moved from the home to the hospital and mothers were alone without family. It is still possible, in a home or hospital, to have a great natural birth.

Currently, in The Bradley Method, 87.7 percent of women having a vaginal birth do so by choice without drugs. Labor and birth is something that can be done by most couples, if they are trained in Bradley classes. Contractions can be very powerful hard work, perhaps the hardest work you have ever done. Women need to know how to get ready for labor and how to handle contractions. Without education and preparation, contractions can be overwhelming.

THE BRADLEY METHOD CLASSES

All Bradley Method classes are twelve weeks long with a curriculum that has worked for hundreds of thousands of couples, and it comes with the current official *The Bradley Method Student Workbook* along with an Official Coach Card.

We have found that we have the highest rate of unmedicated

vaginal births after twelve weeks of preparation with training and education of Mom and Dad. We have found that the rate of medicated births and cesareans rises quickly with fewer than twelve weeks of classes. The human body needs time to prepare for this athletic event.

Attending class one night a week for twelve weeks is a small amount of time to dedicate to this baby, your baby. There is so much to learn, exercises, relaxation, labor rehearsals, nutrition, how to birth, how to coach, etc. The class environment adds to your own self-discipline and confidence. The class adds resources and the experiences of your teachers and fellow classmates. When planning for your baby—take the best classes, twelve weeks is a prudent investment to be well prepared. Classes are cheaper than going to the movies each week, and can be much more rewarding. You will probably spend more money on a car seat than your class series.

LEARNING TO WORK WITH LABOR

Labor is a lot of hard work, and may be felt as pressure, power, or pain. There are several types of pain in birthing. The two most common types of pain in childbirth are good pain and unnecessary pain. Working with contractions makes labor effective. Fighting against contractions makes for unnecessary pain.

"Good pain" comes from hard work or athletic effort. Climbing a mountain or running a race is considered good pain . . . HARD WORK!

"Unnecessary pain" comes from doing things wrong, hurting your body because of lack of knowledge and/or taking unnecessary chances. Fear of pain . . . can lead to chest breathing/hyperventilation (panicky breathing) . . . which then leads to tension . . . building its own pain and panic. This is an escalating cycle.

A third type of pain, rare in childbirth, is "injury pain," which means something really is wrong, or broken. This may require medical attention.

The idea of someone throwing you into ten feet of water at the end of nine months is beyond scary, and if you did not know how to swim you could drown. The same is true in childbirth. You can learn how to give birth, but you need to go to our classes, practice, gain confidence, and be ready for this athletic event.

TIPS ON COACHING CONTRACTIONS

If you and your wife are pregnant and reading this book, you already know lots of ways of handling stress and discomfort. Have you ever stubbed your toe? Have you ever had a headache? No one lives long enough to get pregnant without learning how to handle pain in many ways.

This list comes from couples who shared their favorites with us. Most of them are personal choices and may or may not work for you. Try them out and add your own. Learn more in your Bradley classes.

Coaches, many of these suggestions require active support from you. Be ready and know what to do.

What you need to know is which of these techniques work for you in labor. Make a list of what you have tried before, and what you think would work in labor. Be flexible, women often change their minds during labor.

WAYS OF HANDLING PAIN

(For a complete list refer to The Bradley Method Student Workbook.*)*

Sleep—*A Coaching Responsibility!*
   Lack of sleep can make labor harder.

Abdominal Breathing—*A Coaching Responsibility!*
   Abdominal breathing is normal for human beings. It is
      efficient and effective and conducive to relaxation.

Go to the Bathroom—*A Coaching Responsibility!*
   During labor the body keeps working and the bladder fills

with urine. When the mother goes to the bathroom she will be more comfortable.

Walk It Off—*A Coaching Responsibility!*

Walking in labor can be very pleasant and effective.

Not Lying on the Back—*A Coaching Responsibility!*

Lying on her back can be a problem and can cause unnecessary pain.

Back Rub—*A Coaching Responsibility!*

This is a personal choice and, of course, the dad is the best one suited for this.

Relax—*A Coaching Responsibility!*

Relaxation is the key to labor! When the mother relaxes she is able to let go of her muscles and let the uterus do what it needs to do.

IS THIS REAL LABOR?

Is this really labor? First-time mothers generally ignore or don't feel contractions until a few weeks before birth. Experienced mothers may feel contractions sooner. The question is often, "Is this the real thing?" Dr. Bradley said if you are not sure do five things: (1) eat, (2) drink, (3) walk, (4) bathe or shower, (5) nap. If this is the real thing then labor will continue.

BABIES CAN TRIGGER CONTRACTIONS

You may find it interesting to know that the baby has the ability to cause contractions, and may do so when it feels the need to get out of his environment because he is ready to be born, or perhaps he needs more nourishment because the mother has not had anything to eat or drink recently.

The baby is happy most of the time and has a good time in the uterus. All of his needs are met, and he just grows and floats around in amniotic fluid, playing, kicking, and resting when he wants.

One of the amazing parts of pregnancy is the role of the placenta. It is a flat organ that is attached to the uterus on the mother's side. The baby's side has treelike structures, which channel into the cord that goes to the baby. These treelike structures, or villi, are covered with a membrane covering every branch, so there is a tremendous surface area.

The mother's blood is propelled into the placenta and bathes these structures. At this time the nutrients and oxygen in her blood cross this membrane, going through the umbilical vein to nourish the baby.

In the meantime waste products from the baby return by way of two umbilical arteries, taking the waste products to those treelike structures. The waste products pass through the membrane into the mother's blood—and they are taken way and metabolized by the mother. The blood in the baby is manufactured by the baby, and under normal circumstances there is no crossover of blood from mother to baby (or baby to mother).

The process continues with the mother's blood coming into and out of the placenta— dropping off what the baby needs, and transporting out what the baby is getting rid of. The placenta is an amazing organ, and the only organ of the human body with its own birth, life, and death cycle.

This process continues until the baby is ready to be born, or it feels its needs are not being met. If the mother does not eat, the baby's system says, "Let's make a contraction." The uterus squeezes the placenta and the mother's blood is squished out, and when it relaxes new blood comes in. The baby wants to get nutrients, but if they are not there the baby triggers another contraction.

If the mother doesn't eat because she forgets, or is too busy to eat for the both of them, then the nourishment level drops, and the baby gets worried. Should he stay in and hope Mom eats soon, or should he trigger contractions? These contractions can cause a lot of worry.

When the mother eats, nutrients get into her bloodstream very quickly and when the new blood swishes into the placenta, the baby gets these nutrients and relaxes. It is amazing how many premature labors stop or slow down with a glass of milk and a sandwich. If contractions continue, that is what doctors are for.

COACHES' CHECKLIST FOR FIRST-STAGE LABOR

1. Position

The coach is responsible for the mother's position and environment.

2. Relaxation

The coach is the expert in what relaxation techniques this mother likes.

3. Rub Back

The coach knows which types of rubbing to use.

4. Guide Breathing

If the mother is disrupted, the coach knows how to guide her breathing and get her back on track.

5. Time Contractions

Some mothers appreciate knowing the pattern of labor.

6. Talk to Her

Talking can be relaxing for some women.

WHAT TO DO WHEN PROBLEMS OR QUESTIONS ARISE

First, get more information.

QUESTIONS TO ASK BEFORE GIVING "INFORMED CONSENT"

1. Is the mother okay?
2. Is the baby okay?
3. What is the problem?
4. What are we afraid might happen?
5. If we choose this procedure or drug(s), what other things will be necessary?
6. How much time do we have?
7. Could this be normal?
8. What other choices do we have?

These are a few of the tips that are covered in depth in your Bradley class.

THE CESAREAN EPIDEMIC

Most women start labor with a plan of having a natural, unmedicated birth. Often complications, interventions, lack of preparation and confidence make it necessary to change their plans. Some women choose to have a cesarean even though it introduces the risks of major surgery for mother and baby! Medical intervention and cesarean surgery may be appropriate in rare instances to save lives.

Cesarean sections are on the rise today. In the United States we have a 31.1 percent C-section rate, and it has been climbing every year! Over one million cesareans will be performed this year. The C-section rate remains more than twice what experts advise. This means that over half a million unnecessary cesareans are being done each year. This is an epidemic!

SIX LEADING CAUSES OF CESAREANS
- Inability to relax
- CPD (cephalo-pelvic-disproportion, too small a pelvic opening)
- Failure to progress (dilate) rapidly
- Fetal distress
- Prolonged labor
- Pain, fear, fatigue

Women can prepare and help themselves!

BENEFITS OF PREGNANCY EXERCISES IN AVOIDING A CESAREAN

Is it possible a few simple exercises could help women avoid cesarean sections?

The following exercises address what many experts feel are

the six leading causes of cesarean surgery. Many pregnant women have told us that by preparing ahead of time they were ready for labor. These exercises and relaxation practices are most effective if practiced on a daily basis for at least three months before birth. Check with your doctor before starting any exercise program. Your Bradley instructor will teach you how in class.

PELVIC ROCK

This is a wonderful exercise that gently tones and conditions the mother's abdominal muscles in a way that encourages the baby into a good position, possibly reducing the chances of a cesarean section. This exercise also helps deal with back pain and encourages a posterior baby to turn naturally for an easier birth.

KEGELS

Having done this exercise will help keep the baby's chin on its chest, as it begins its journey through the pelvis. This makes a big difference in the size of the presenting part.

WALKING

Walking opens the inlet of the pelvis, which encourages the baby to come down. It speeds labor on an average of 28 percent. It reduces the amount of pain mothers experience in labor and reduces the likelihood that a mother will need an epidural (which itself may lead to a cesarean).

SIDE-LYING POSITION

Gives mothers a comfortable alternative to the traditional flat-on-the-back position, which is known to cause fetal distress. Lying on the back can also cause an incredible amount of totally unnecessary pain, prolonged labor, and failure to progress.

SQUATTING

Squatting during pregnancy helps to prepare the pelvis for birth, reducing CPD. During second stage (expulsion) this position increases the outlet of the pelvis by more than 10 percent.

Just imagine how many cesareans this exercise alone could prevent!

THINGS TO REMEMBER . . .

This is the birth of your baby, no matter how it is born. There are special things you should remember, write in the baby's book, and tell your Bradley teacher about.

1. What did the baby look like the first time you saw him/her?
2. What was the baby's color . . . pink from the start? bluish? How soon did your baby pink up?
3. What did the baby's eyes look like . . . alert, sleepy? Did you look into your baby's eyes at birth?
4. What did the baby feel like the first time you touched him/her? Wet, dry, smooth?
5. What did the baby smell like? There is a newborn human smell!
6. Did the baby have hair? What color? Wet or dry? Short or long?
7. How soon did the baby respond to your touch or voice?

Take pictures and write your observations and thoughts down. Ask the mother the same things. This is what you want to remember: the baby, and the joy of seeing your baby come into the world . . . no matter how it is born.

FINAL THOUGHTS

Natural childbirth is an athletic, learned experience. Families can learn how to give birth naturally and bond the family unit even closer than before. Other mammals learn about birth from one another in their environment. Humans can learn from experienced teachers in a class environment. The Bradley Method classes meet for twelve weeks to give you time to become skilled at pregnancy, exercises, and labor rehearsals. Many couples take The Bradley Method childbirth classes because they want to learn how to give birth naturally, avoiding unnecessary drugs and cesareans. Classes cover a series of topics: some simple exercises, lots of in-class relaxation, weekly nutrition logs, many labor rehearsals, and more.

Dr. Bradley was fond of saying, "A husband should be man enough to finish what he starts!" Thank you for caring enough to be there for such a wonderful, life-altering experience!

INDEX

ABOUT THE AUTHORS

Robert A. Bradley, M.D. (1917–1998), began practicing and promoting the principles of true natural childbirth in 1947, and wrote the first edition of this book in 1965. He devoted himself full-time to the general practice in obstetrics and gynecology in Denver for several decades. At the time of his death in 1998, The Bradley Method had directly affected more than half a million births.

The American Academy of Husband-Coached Childbirth was cofounded by Dr. Bradley and executive directors Marjie and Jay Hathaway, who live in southern California and have traveled the country training Bradley teachers since 1970. Together with their son, James (vice president of the Academy), they have updated and expanded this revised edition.